ON
HAVING A
Heart Attack

Also by William O'Rourke

The Harrisburg 7 and the New Catholic Left

The Meekness of Isaac

On the Job: Fiction about Work by Contemporary American Writers (editor)

Idle Hands

Criminal Tendencies

Signs of the Literary Times: Essays, Reviews, Profiles, 1970–1992

Notts

Campaign America '96: The View from the Couch

Campaign America 2000: The View from the Couch

ON
HAVING A
Heart Attack

A MEDICAL MEMOIR

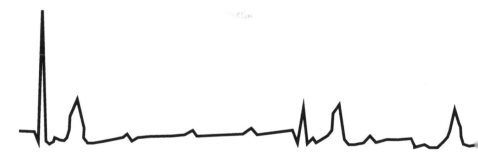

William O'Rourke

UNIVERSITY OF NOTRE DAME PRESS

NOTRE DAME, INDIANA

I would like to thank the editors of the *Indy Men's Magazine* and *Perfect 10*,
where portions of this book appeared in different form.

The cardiac catheterization diagram (Figure A) is reproduced courtesy of
Ronald D. Nelson, M.D.

Library of Congress Cataloging in-Publication Data
O'Rourke, William.
On having a heart attack : a medical memoir / William O'Rourke.
p.   cm.
Includes bibliographical references.
ISBN-13: 978-0-268-03726-0 (cloth : alk. paper)
ISBN-10: 0-268-03726-4 (cloth : alk. paper)
1. O'Rourke, William—Health.   2. Myocardial infarction—Patients—
United States—Biography.   3. Myocardial infarction—Patients—United
States—Rehabilitation.   I. Title.
RC685.I6079 2006
362.196'12370092—dc22

                                                    2006000832

TO
Joseph

Contents

A Note to the Reader

Cardiovascular disease is the leading cause of morbidity and mortality in the United States, responsible for almost 50 percent of all deaths. More than 13.5 million Americans have a history of myocardial infarction or experience angina pectoris. Nearly 1.5 million Americans sustain myocardial infarction each year, of which almost 500,000 are fatal. Five percent of myocardial infarctions occur in people younger than age 40, and about 45 percent occur in people under age 65.
—Cardiac Rehabilitation, Clinical Guideline No. 17, 1995

Our own medical knowledge and practice give us a different relation to both. Very crudely, the fact that we can keep alive people who would then have died means that we are familiar with chronic states in a way [earlier generations] were not.
—Ruth Padel, *Whom Gods Destroy*

What follows is an account of one man's heart attack. My own. Following my heart attack, I read a great deal of the literature about the subject and discovered many things: One thing I found lacking in the available books were descriptions of the heart attack itself, as well as the hospitalization that follows. The former seemed to occupy but a paragraph or two, the latter a few pages at most.

There weren't many accounts by patients on having heart attacks available in the 1990s. A friend, Emily Jane Goodman, wrote a moving account of her husband's heart attack and its treatment for *New York* magazine in 1988, and there are other accounts by spouses and bystanders, as well as many books by doctors about how to avoid heart attacks and how to live beyond them. And there are books about bypass surgeries, both before and after, or previous to, a heart attack. Geoffrey Wolff wrote a generally humorous essay about his heart troubles, a "valve job," in his book *A Day at the Beach.* All of these have something to offer (a good many of them are listed in the bibliography). There is even a subset of health literature, books by doctors themselves who contract some disease or condition. It is hard to keep a pen from those trained hands, it appears.

To remedy the lack in the literature I offer a far more extended look at having a heart attack, what the experience feels like, and what people around the patient tend to do about it—from a patient's point of view.

The first chapter of the book covers the heart attack itself and the next three continue with the subsequent hospitalization. I then deal with the pre– and post–heart attack world I was in—and remain in. Indeed, in a few instances, I recount what is occurring in the present tense, so present it remains to me. Additionally, you will find a good deal of information about treatment and prevention in the main text and the notes, and in the back matter.

One of the handful of volumes by a patient about having a heart attack is Norman Cousins's *The Healing Heart,* published in 1983. Times change. And one large change is that my book is not written with the same sort of triumphalism that Cousins employs. Indeed, my story is both pessimistic and optimistic. I am not a drum beater for the powers of positive thinking. (Cousins is famously known not for his heart book, but for an earlier one about a different malady, *Anatomy of an Illness.*) Cousins's situation was unique, since he was a non-physician teaching in a medical school at the time of his heart attack. And, because of that, the quality and amount of medical attention lavished upon Cousins are quite stunning. What I recount herein is the more ordinary experience, the one, for good or ill, most people will encounter. But it has lessons too. If forewarned is forearmed, you will profit from knowing what I—belatedly—know. And if you, too, have survived an MI (myocardial infarction, the medical term for a heart attack), I hope you'll find some comfort and recognition in the pages beyond.

I didn't have a large appetite for self-help books before I had my heart attack (not enough salt and fat in their makeup, I suppose). But I would like to think this book is the sort of self-help book I would have read, had it been available: personal, informative, literate, the average experience. This, however, is a medical memoir, not a full memoir. I only make use of my life as it seems to bear on the heart attack itself.

At this point, I would like to offer some acknowledgments. The following provided aid and comfort in a variety of ways during the period of my heart attack and during the writing of this book: my wife, Teresa Ghilarducci, and my son, Joe; the doctors—especially Drs. Vinod Chauhan, John Kobayashi, and Ronald Nelson—and nurses and staff at St. Joseph's Hospital and Cardiology Associates in South Bend, Indiana; my parents and brothers and sisters; my colleagues at the University of Notre Dame; my agent, Linda Roghaar; and the specific following individuals, in alphabetical order: Dorothy Baker, Matt Benedict, Bill Binder, David Black, Joe Blenkinsopp, Susan Blum, Robert Burke, Ford Burkhart, Kevin Coyne, Charles DeFanti, Corinne Demas, Margaret Doody, John Duffy, Chris Fox, Judy Fox, Dolores Frese, Jerry Frese, David Ghilarducci, M.D., Sally Ghilarducci, Joan Harris, Lou Harry, David Hoppe, Thomas A. Hughes, M.D., Chris Jara, Lionel Jensen, Tom Kapacinskas, Robert Kareka, Zane Kotker, David Matlin, John Matthias, Marsha McCreadie, Jay Neugeboren, Jerome Neyrey, S.J., Craig Nova, John O'Brien, Jean Porter, Judith Robert, Keith Russell, Nettie Russell, Valerie Sayers, Betty Signer, Michael Signer, Janey Skeer, Roger Skillings, Irini Spanidou, Mark Stanish, M.D., John Wright Stevens, Chris Tiedemann, Ed Zuckerman.

CHAPTER ONE

Here's Mine

I was home in South Bend, Indiana, in my attic office, working on a novel involving coal miners, set against the backdrop of the 1984–85 National Union of Miners strike in England. The phone rang, and it was Eric Sandeen, the oldest child of my friends Eileen and Ernie Sandeen. Eric, a professor of American Studies at the University of Wyoming, was in town to go to the Notre Dame–University of Southern California football game. His father was an emeritus professor of English at Notre Dame, and Eric was using his tickets. He had an extra one for the game that was to start in about an hour, and he offered it to me. I had donated my tickets to some good cause. It was October 26, 1991, and the fall weather was only fair, but the gray, overcast sky wasn't supposed to turn into rain.

My day's work of writing was about over, in any case: the cold, wet atmosphere of the novel's English pit towns had seeped into me, and the change of location, of the chance to go outside, was appealing. My novel, for a number of reasons, had been hard going. I decided to abandon it and attend the game.

I went downstairs and told my wife I was leaving. She was working at her computer, preparing testimony for an appearance as an expert witness (she is an economist), and she looked at me skeptically but bid me adieu. She said, "I'm so worried about Monday, my heart hurts."

Our fifteen-month-old, Joe, was downstairs with Maria, a baby-sitter we had retained for three hours so both my wife and I could get some work done. Eric was impatient to get into the stadium (he was an alum and wanted to bask in the pregame show); I was in a rush to get there, to try not to delay him any further.

The coal miners of Great Britain would have to wait. I said good-bye to everyone in the house and took off. What going to the game meant was that Teresa would have to take care of Joe by herself after Maria left. I had planned to watch the game on television, which would have left me able to look after Joe. We were attempting to divide looking after our boy 50/50, which in these modern co-parenting arrangements amounted to doing it 75/75. Teresa's father had been an all-American football player at Berkeley, but she was not a fan. Football was the bane of fall weekends for her as a new mother—as it was when she was a young girl.

We lived near the campus, but on a football weekend the university becomes a sports franchise. To get to the closest parking available required a circuitous route through South Bend's downtown and then approaching the campus obliquely from the south, parking in a poor neighborhood adjacent to the campus.

South Bend isn't a college town, and the university always has been separate from it, especially back in the heyday of the city, when the Studebaker car company was South Bend's major employer. But now Notre Dame is the largest employer, and, though the campus is still on the town's northern edge, the school is central to the business interests here. I parked my old Volvo near Notre Dame Avenue, by the house I owned when I first moved to town, about four blocks from campus.

At the time, it was a neighborhood of student rentals, African American households, and a few junior faculty, which is what I had been when I lived there. Notre Dame Avenue is a broad street that goes straight into the heart of the campus. It is wide because there are railroad tracks beneath layers of asphalt, tracks of the South Shore railroad; in the halcyon days of the early and mid twentieth century, the era of Ronald Reagan as the Gipper, the South Shore Line used to come into the campus, as well as travelling straight through the middle of downtown South Bend.

After parking, I walked quickly to the stadium. It was about a half hour before kickoff. There were stragglers on the periphery of the campus, but most of the 60,000 people were either in or around the stadium, tailgating in the pay parking lots, swarming around the brick edges of the stadium like ants around a morsel. I met Eric beneath the entrance he specified, and he gave me a ticket. It was a good seat, better than my own season tickets provided.

Eric rushed in, and I told him I'd join him after I got something at the concession stand. I hadn't eaten lunch, so I wanted a hot dog. I stood in line, put in my order for a Polish kielbasa, the thicker sort of hot dog, and a Diet Coke.

As I walked away with my refreshments, I felt something peculiar. It was so strange it stopped me mid-step. I was forty-five years old, and I had felt many things, but never before this particular feeling: I felt a click deep inside. The image the sensation produced in my mind was of a BB, a small round piece of copper-colored lead, falling into a socket. It was a very clear image. A BB is tiny, but the one I imagined felt infinitesimal, microscopic. Yet I felt it, a click, metal on metal—like an expensive, microscopic gear had slipped, some exquisite piece of machinery falling out of alignment. Some medieval example of craftsmanship, a gyroscope, something intricate, needing fine balance. The feeling, the event, was located in my chest, below my left breast. It was thoroughly interior, as if a signal had been sent and registered, what those giant satellite dishes are poised waiting for, a transmission from deep space.

I continued on into the stadium to find my seat and join Eric. They were great seats, practically on the fifty-yard line. And they were real seats, with backs, not just a slab of lumber to sit on as I was used to, and we were only a few rows from the field.

The seat was so good someone was sitting in it—a woman, it turned out, who had misread her ticket's row number. After she moved, I sat down and thought about eating my large hot dog. But I began to feel sick to my stomach. Since I hadn't eaten for a few hours, I couldn't understand why. But I did feel nauseous. So much so I put my head between my legs to bring myself some comfort, to get some blood to my head, I supposed. Then I felt something electric, part tingle, part buzz, traveling down through my left arm.

I'm not sure how long I was bent over. I heard Eric say something along the lines of, "Are you all right?"

I replied, "I'm not sure." I began to feel cold and clammy.

I jerked myself up. It seemed that the temperature had dropped thirty degrees. My shoulders were up and my neck compressed down as if I were freezing. The electric feeling in my arm was creeping up my shoulder into my neck. I felt sweaty. I looked at my right hand. It was blazingly white. My left hand still had the hot dog in it, wrapped in tin foil. I put the hot dog in the pocket of my coat.

I heard Eric then say, from what sounded like a long way away, "Do you think it has to do with your heart?" I heard that, but I didn't react to it. It was as if I saw someone I thought I knew, but couldn't actually remember who it was. The question just hung there.

I am not sure how much time had passed. Three minutes? Five? But it took me at least that long to admit to myself what was going on. I was having a heart attack. I had read and heard the list of symptoms enough times. It seemed a classic case. Nausea, tingling in the arm, sweat. The tightness of my neck and shoulders. I considered none of it pain: I had been hurtled forward into another state, one I had never been in, as if I were in outer space without a suit.

I knew there was a first aid station in the stadium. I needed to get there, but I didn't know where it was located in relation to these unfamiliar seats. I looked about and there seemed to be a mist in the stadium, a fog, one that transmitted color. Some USC players were on the field in front of me; they moved slowly, silently. The gold and red of their uniforms glowed incandescently.

I swung my head back around and looked for an usher. He would know. I told Eric I was going to the first aid station, and I heard him get up behind me. There, at the end of the row, was a frail old man with an usher's cap on. He must be near ninety, I thought. I asked him where the first aid station was, and he looked at me with concern and took my arm and led me through a tunnel to the concourse below the stands. This was familiar. I did not resist his help, though I thought it must look strange, a man twice my age helping me along. People parted before us, rubbernecking pedestrians, most staring with curiosity and alarm. Just who looked older or more frail at that moment, me or the usher, I cannot say.

Even in my distress, I thought us a strange sight, though I had seen one dying person walking before. It was 1981, and I was visiting my closest friends, Robert and Inez Kareka in Boston, right before I came out to the Midwest to start teaching at Notre Dame.

Inez had been fighting cancer for two years, and her battle was almost over. In the middle of the night noise had awakened me. I saw Robert helping Inez to the bathroom. She had been asleep in the living room and had opened the refrigerator door, thinking it was the bathroom and had backed into it, crashing its contents. He was leading Inez to the actual bathroom, and she looked transformed; she was in her late fifties then and had always been a looker, in the style of Marilyn Monroe, of whose generation she was.

But that night her dyed blonde hair was wildly askew. Her hair's black roots framed her thinned face, her now stick-like limbs were held akimbo, and her expression was fixed in a muted scream, as if she wanted to say something but had lost the language to do so. She looked like a Goya etching. And that morning she went into a coma she never came out of until she died a week later.

In the stadium, as I dragged my legs and waved my arms as I walked along with the ancient usher, I thought I, too, must look like death.

We got to the door of the first aid station, and, as we entered, the silence that had seemed to surround me vanished. There was a TV on tuned to the pregame show. People were animated, talking. Eric stayed by the door.

"Is there a doctor here?" I asked. A few people in the room came toward me quickly. "Here, get his coat off." I was wearing an expensive Barbour coat I had bought in England. It had the hot dog in the pocket. I sat down, and someone began to unbutton my shirt. Another hand had grabbed my wrist, and I heard a voice say, "I can't find a pulse."

He said it to a slightly older man, but not that much older than I. "Oh, you're probably just hyperventilating," the man who was addressed said to me.

He must be the doctor, I thought. "I'm a professor here," I said. "I've taught for over ten years, and I've never hyperventilated in my life. If I'm hyperventilating, put a bag over my head."

No one was going to say what was obvious: He's having a heart attack. Not even I. But I did feel better that I was saying something forceful, that I had some force. Eric (who is very tall) was looming by the doorway. The doctor said, We'll get you to the hospital just to be safe. There was more motion around the room. Eric said something about going to the hospital with me, and I said, No, stay, enjoy the game. He had come a long way to go to the game. I thought I heard him say he would call Teresa.

My shirt hung, unbuttoned, loose around me. My coat was gone. A gurney was produced near the doorway, and I was led to it and helped up to lie down on it. Straps were put over me, and I was wheeled down the concourse. I was now staring upward at the concrete rafters and would glimpse the occasional face looking down at me, again with a mixture of alarm, curiosity, and concern. I was a spectacle. The game hadn't yet begun. An ambulance was parked near one of the stadium's gates. I had seen it there before and took little notice. The gurney's legs were collapsed, and it was picked up by two men wearing similar coats and rolled into the ambulance. One of the men hopped into the ambulance's narrow cabin and began to attempt to put an IV into the skin above my left hand. They wanted to drip something in. He kept sticking me, trying to get a good purchase on a vein, but seemed not to be having much luck. His attempts didn't hurt. I seemed to have a surface numbness. I was just unhappy he wasn't succeeding. It seemed as if a lot of time were passing and nothing were going on. Finally, he stopped trying and left the needle inserted in whatever fashion it was and taped it. More minutes seemed to pass, and finally the doors of the ambulance closed.

I could picture where the ambulance was going, after it finally started to move. Though I was wearing a watch, I wasn't looking at it. Time was both elongated and slowed. Here was the now; I was in it. The ambulance needed to part the waters; there were still crowds around the stadium, and there was no direct way out. It twisted and turned, and finally I felt it speed up as it hit city streets. It turned out they were going straight up Notre Dame Avenue. Lying down on the gurney, I was a mass of resistance; my shoulders continued to rise, as my neck and head attempted to retract into my body, turtle-like. The sensation in my arm and neck was no longer an electrical buzz; it was molecular, an ethereal feeling, as if I were being transported somewhere—and not just my body being ferried in an ambulance. Its siren was on, but it didn't seem loud. Turning my head, I saw the roof of my former house go by; here, literally, was my life passing by. But what I was feeling was the sense of being erased. As if I were a stone on the surface of the water, about to be swallowed over, rippleless. I felt, as clearly as I have ever felt anything, how everything in the world would go on without me.

Here and gone. Gone gone gone. Then, what I knew surfaced, how this ride up the empty street (because of the game there was no traffic on it) was so much like all the mythology I had ever read: Lethe, the river Styx, the voyage across, death's boatman, Charon at the wheel, the trip to Elysium. In the eerie quiet of the ambulance I was being taken away. Away. The ferry men were riding up front. I was alone.

We arrived at the hospital. Doors opened, and I was rolled out and in, ending up in an examining room, one of the ambulance attendants carrying the drip that he had attempted to hook up to me. I heard him say to a nurse he didn't think it was right. I was still on my back. A nurse took my hand and prepared another intravenous line. She left in the one he had inserted. Another drip was started through the new one.

Someone asked, "Are you from out of town?"

It seemed an odd question. Beyond the drip that had been started, nothing was happening. I was prone, making sounds that were between language and a moan.

I thought then of what they were looking at: A short, overweight, white male in his mid forties, with thinning hair, without a prosperous-looking face. I was wearing old work shoes, from Sears Roebuck, "Die Hard" (!) embossed on their soles. Khaki pants that were close to twenty years old, as was the old, worn leather belt. The flannel shirt hanging loosely on me, though not twenty years old, was frayed and old enough.

"I'm a professor at Notre Dame," I said weakly.

I didn't hear a harrumph, but no one said anything. There continued to be some milling about. I lay there thinking someone should be doing something.

"I'm a professor at Notre Dame," I repeated more forcefully to no discernible effect.

Time passed, too much time, I thought and, with some difficulty, I got myself to sit up, and, with my right arm and hand, the one that wasn't singing with molecular activity and didn't have a drip inserted into it, I awkwardly fished for my wallet. I laid it open on my thigh and slowly thumbed through the contents till I found the thin and shiny BlueCross card. I waved it above my head.

"Here's my insurance card," I proclaimed.

It was snatched from my hand, and the room was immediately transformed into a beehive of activity. My shirt was removed, an oxygen necklace was draped around my face. I was given nitroglycerin to take under my tongue, and someone appeared with a clipboard to take more information. Questions were asked, names, addresses. An EKG machine was wheeled in, and I was hooked up to it. An intravenous line was inserted into my other hand.

I realized that had I been wearing my English Barbour waxed jacket, someone would have recognized it as the costly thing it was, and made some judgment other than that I might be a derelict. I felt whatever had caused the inactivity was my appearance; I did not appear to be a man of substance until I produced my Blue Cross card.

Finally, someone I took to be a doctor came into the room; she appeared to be in her late twenties, dark-haired with a good haircut, thin, and she had a stethoscope hung around her neck. She looked at the EKG printout and wandered out of the room.

I was still sitting up in my parody of a freezing posture, shoulder blades peaked, neck squashed, and I noticed I was talking out loud to myself. I was saying what I was thinking. As if I thought I couldn't hear myself think and needed to say it out loud. Then, out loud, I asked, "Why am I talking to myself out loud?" And I answered myself, "Because I'm scared."

The doctor walked back into the room. She didn't react to what I had been saying, though I wanted her to join the conversation, so I asked, "Did the EKG show any heart involvement?" Not waiting for an answer, I said, "The doctor earlier at the stadium said he thought I was hyperventilating." Why I was still offering that bit of wishful thinking, I don't know, but I presume it had to do with being scared. She responded with only one word, "Yes," and I knew it was the answer to the heart question. "You should try to relax," she said, and walked out again.

Relax! Are you nuts? I thought, but, this time, didn't say aloud. She had said it reproachfully, standing a few feet from me. Oh, sure, I'm going to try to relax. I'm having a heart attack. If I could make my shoulders look less like Mount Kilimanjaro, I would. Relax.

I was being silent, though, not talking aloud to myself anymore.

An old man appeared at the door, wearing what looked like a highway hazard jacket, as if he were in the street, directing traffic. He was as old as the usher and looked like there might be a family resemblance, which made his orange and red fright jacket seem even more incongruous.

"Your son is out in the waiting room and wants to see you," he said.

"Ahhh," I wailed. "He can't be out there! It's not my son. He's only fifteen months old!"

I felt as if I were keening, though I'm not sure what it sounded like. A sorrow deeper than despair hit me. I wondered if I was hallucinating. My son was waiting for me. For a fleeting second I wondered if that could possibly be true. Had Eric called anyone? Hadn't I asked him to call Teresa? Didn't he volunteer?

Nonetheless, I felt overcome, but I swallowed the sob. I was born. I finally had a child, a son. Then I died. My job was done.

A nurse wheeled in another bag, fussed with the intravenous line, attached an access joint to it, and began another drip. "Morphine," she said. "That should help."

As I tried not to think about my son waiting outside for me, I realized I should call Teresa. The doctor had come back into the room (doubtless to see if I had "relaxed") and had again turned her back to me while looking at some papers.

"Could you call my wife, please? And tell her I'm here," I said, and told her the number. The doctor complied, and I heard her speak softly into the receiver, though I couldn't make out the words. The hospital was less than ten minutes from our home.

I was breathing the fresh oxygen, thinking it must be for my brain cells. I continued to remain upright, and I wondered what the morphine was doing to me, for me. I didn't feel any pain. Morphine was for pain, wasn't it?

I was already feeling utterly transformed, pushed into another dimension, a state hitherto unknown. Pain, in my lexicon, was being sliced by glass, or some other such calamity. No, I wasn't in pain. I was somewhere else. Not ecstasy, certainly. But I realized I was beginning to feel somewhat out of body: *ex stasis*. Looking down on myself. Perhaps, I thought, that's why people who are near death often report themselves floating around, looking at the operating table or people in the room. That must be the morphine, I considered. I seemed to be disassociating. I still wasn't sure how much time had passed, but too much, I thought, without something crucial happening.

Then I saw my wife rush by the doorway and start to come back toward it, when she was intercepted by the doctor. The doctor was telling her, "You've got to get him to relax." That I heard very clearly. The relaxation cure.

My wife walked into the room, her brown eyes wide.

"I'm hyperventilating," I said. "They say I'm hyperventilating."

Why I offered her the same nonsense the first aid room doctor offered me, I don't know. Then I said, much more to the point, "I'm sorry."

She knew what I was sorry for. I was sorry for having a heart attack.

"They want you to relax."

"I know. I'm trying," I said, knowing I wasn't succeeding.

I was expecting her to come up to me, to touch me. But, at first, she stayed in the same spot the doctor had occupied, near the wall, near a counter, as if a magnet held people there. Or, perhaps, the sight of me created a force field. Looking at someone having a heart attack mustn't be attractive. It would have been reassuring to be touched, other than to have needles inserted. She finally came forward and grasped my ankle; my legs were the only extremities without tubes or wires attached. But that kept her a few feet from me. It still felt as if it were thirty below all around me.

It must have been at least an hour since I felt the click, the tiny ball falling out of the socket. It became clear that everyone must be waiting for something, and it wasn't for me to start relaxing. A doctor. They were waiting for a Doctor, capital D. The young woman must be an intern. Do heart attacks just go on and on? That was frightening, though I was already past frightened. Physically, the morphine wasn't making the sensations I felt any different, except that I seemed to continue to separate from them. My consciousness had become slippery.

My wife and the young doctor (whom I had turned into an intern) were conferring again in the hallway. A nurse came in and adjusted the drips (which I later learned were Lidocaine and heparin). And the oxygen. I had been given nitroglycerin under my tongue, but I wasn't sure of its effects. I knew it was standard. I was given more.

My wife was telling someone that I had just walked a couple miles with her the day before and hadn't been short of breath.

I hadn't ever experienced any angina. I didn't know what angina felt like, since I never had it. It seemed, given the questions, some sort of decision remained, loomed, needed to be made.

The clot of people in the hallway thickened. I realized it had been all female, and now there was a male. After the ambulance duo had left, and the odd ancient messenger looking for some son's father, everyone in attendance had been female. The new arrival, Dr. V. C., was male, short, dark-haired, thin.

A great time to have a heart attack. Early Saturday afternoon. Where were all the cardiologists? On the golf course? At the game? I now realized that when I had answered earlier the question of who my doctor was, and had given the name of my allergist, that had been important information. They must have tried to contact him first, I presumed, some chain of command, responsibility, protocol, the land of referrals. Who was going to take charge? It appeared to me it was this guy, standing next to me, asking me what happened. I knew it was a test: of lucidity, of my condition, my state. And what I said might have something to do with what he chose to do next.

I was at the football game, I told him, and then was hit with symptoms—nausea, tightness, odd feelings in my arm, up to my neck, clammy, sweat. I got to the first aid station, was told I was hyperventilating, was taken to the hospital; here I am. My wife was listening too; most of it was news to her. The doctor seemed satisfied. He said to increase the amount of morphine I was getting and, once more, that I should try to relax. And that I should be administered tPA, a clot-busting drug.

"Do you have it?" he asked. "Is it prepared? A bolus." I fastened on that word, since it was from a different vocabulary, a medical term. I began to picture a bolus, a golf-ball size something, another sphere, shiny, silver, bigger than a BB. My wife was quizzing him on what it was: the tPA may eat through the clot that was causing the heart attack. I caught that much. The morphine was messing with my concentration.

Time passed, clipboards were consulted, the bolus was prepared. Finally, a nurse came in with a hypodermic. The doctor said, "All right. Give it to him." It was said casually, but the folk in the room had seemed to have acquired my tenseness. Now, everyone had become stiff. The nurse inserted the needle into a junction in the tube and delivered the hypodermic's contents into the IV, which then flowed into me.

The doctor, responding to a question from my wife, had told her that the tPA had a 60 percent chance of breaking up the clot.

"You mean," she said, alarmed, "it has a 40 percent chance of not working?"

She is an economist. A scientist. They call economics the dismal science, and that was a dismal statistic. There was a bustle of hands around me. I was to be taken up to cardiac intensive care.

I was now reclining, and someone was pushing the gurney out the room's door. A blonde nurse was standing nearby; I had noticed her earlier: she had not done much so far but had reacted to other people's remarks and had seemed the most emotional of the nurses, because she had actually showed some emotion, an underlying discontent, a kind of anger—she seemed to be mad at the heart attack itself, what it was doing to me. She touched me on the arm and said as I was wheeled off, "Did anyone tell you that it will hurt more if that works?"

No, I said, knowing what "that works" meant. The tPA. She seemed to be telling me a secret or, at least, the truth.

⌁The clanking, the rolling, the filling of the elevator occur, and I am taken upstairs, moved ("one, two, three, lift") onto a hospital bed. The drips are rearranged. The room has monitors, chairs, a television suspended, curtains that can be drawn around the bed. It is a single. It doesn't seem brightly lit; gray light comes in through a window. Transferred to a bed, lying down, I hope the morphine is working without my realizing it. But I feel under pressure, as if I am going to explode; it's a kind of writhing.

I finally realize what that means: the body writhes. I am moaning. My wife is standing near the foot of the bed. I can see her. There are a couple of nurses, both female. No one who appears to be a doctor has come along. Nurses say things, but my concentration is shattered. A nurse is applying cold compresses, wet washcloths, to my forehead, as if we're in a Western at the turn of the twentieth century and there is nothing to do but apply a damp cloth for comfort.

I bolt upright.

"Now this hurts," I say aloud. The force of the experience has lifted me off the bed."Ah."

I think that "this" can't continue, whatever it is I'm feeling. Nothing before would I have called pain, but this is intolerable. It is as if I am being burnt alive while hurtling through space. I expect some reaction from the women around me, my wife, but they just stare. How long can this go on?

"Ahhh," I let out again, and drop backwards onto the bed.

It's over.[1]

Slowly, it dawns on me: I now feel as I felt before I walked up to the concession stand to buy my hot dog. All at once, it seems that the drugs I've been given for the past hour or so take effect instantaneously, as if I have been suspended over a pool of morphine, held up above its surface by the thin wire of the heart attack, and the wire has snapped. And I feel myself falling into the silvery water, submerging, warmth around me. I pass out.

CHAPTER TWO

Connected to Time

My connection to time still hasn't completely reestablished itself, but I can feel myself gliding up toward consciousness. The room isn't empty. I make out that my wife is there and there is a man standing next to her. I'm not wearing my glasses, and their two bodies are just forms, shapes in a mist.

I hear the man say, "Is he your father?"

"No," I hear my wife say, "he's my husband."

The man's shape becomes darker: a black suit, a collar. He's a priest, I assume.

I slip back into unconsciousness.

─⋁─ When I awake again the room is bright. Lights are on. I am amazed at how I feel. It is no longer thirty below. I am still wired up. I can see my heart rate numbers and an oscillating wave, a green line, spiking up and down, not flat. I am being fussed over by a nurse. I ask for water.

─⋁─ Later, my wife appears at the door of the room, holding our son, Joe. She holds him up high, so he can see above the equipment surrounding the bed. Joe looks worried, almost frantic; he turns his head this way and that.

"Hi, sweetie," I say. I wave at him awkwardly, with my hands stuck with IVs.

"We can't stay," my wife says. "They don't want him to be here."

"OK," I say. "I'm all right, Joe. See you soon. I love you."

They disappear from the doorway. They were there, I assure myself.

I begin to consider Teresa's problems: babysitters, the absence of. Co-parenting put on hold. She is teaching; I am on leave. She would have to work things out. I tried to remember if I had been away from Joe since he was born. My wife travels a lot; I don't. But now I was gone, in the hospital. On a weekend. Was today Sunday? Still Saturday?

—⋀— Nothing much seems to happen over the weekend in a hospital. Some visits blur together. A number of doctors see me. The first, my wife and son's doctor, E. S., came by. She said she looked at my chart and things appeared to be fairly good. She mentioned some reading that gave an indication of heart damage. But very little, she said.

The next doctor I saw was Dr. V. C., the cardiologist who had ordered the bolus of tPA. He said he looked at my chart and it didn't look too good. I protested. What? Earlier I had just heard the opposite.

No, he said, the readings were bad.

My wife arrived.[1] I reported the little knowledge I had, although, thus far, good or bad didn't have much geography for me. I didn't know the landscape, the distance between good and bad. Just then, Dr. V. C. returned and said, sheepishly, Yes, the results weren't so bad after all. He said he had read the chart wrong; he had read it upside down.

After he—a bit chastened—left, Teresa said, "Well, it took something to come in and admit that." The news cheered me up, sort of.

Two other doctors visited. One I had gone to for my allergies when I first moved to Indiana. After decades of sneezing and watery eyes, I finally discovered one could (might) do something about that. Also, I had health coverage. He had trained as an internist (he told me the story of his arrival in Indiana one summer: seeing all the fields of corn, soybeans, pollen-producing crops, had told him he had come to the right place, a bonanza for allergists). My allergist/internist seemed a very hyper guy to me, high strung, but my allergies got better. For the last few years he had considered putting me on blood pressure medicine, but each time he decided to see if the effects of diet and exercise would lower it. After a few years of sporadic diet and exercise, my blood pressure (and weight) was still high.

So his visit was rather melancholy, but I didn't feel much like blaming him. He wanted to hand me off to a new internist, which seemed like the thing to do. I tried to think of an analogy for that (changing agents, publishers?). Changing driving instructors after a car crash came the closest, I thought.

The new doctor appeared, a slightly younger man (though my internist was younger than I was), very neat, wearing a new L. L. Bean windbreaker. OK, I'd be seeing him. They both worked at the same clinic.

But I had also gained a group of cardiologists, the group the first doctor worked with. I had begun to piece together what the group's structure was. The doctor who had been dragged in on Saturday was the electrical man: He did pacemakers and heart-related circuitry. I would be seeing the group's plumber soon. They wanted to do tests: an angiogram and perhaps an angioplasty.[2] The vocabulary that may have flown around my head in the past had now landed on my shoulders. There were other specialties, if it came to that. The reconstructionists, the bypass people.

I finally heard what sounded like a diagnosis. I had "hemorrhaged into plaque." That was to become a familiar utterance.

My wife had called my parents, and they said they were coming. She hadn't asked them to, but it would lessen some of her difficulties and take care of the babysitting problem.

⌁ For dinner I am served a pork chop. Somewhere it says I am on a low-salt diet, but I wonder what the pork chop qualifies as. It does recall my parents to me, who are arriving today. The hospital pork chop looks like the ones my mother served one night a week every week of my childhood, though hers had more fat around the edges. Beyond that succulence, they had the shape and feel of a shoe heel. This one too, except there is little fat on it—the only thing with taste. My height and weight are up on a dry board. Five foot five, which is an inch short, I felt, and 203 pounds—which must be about ten too many, I tell myself.

I think about when I gained my extra weight and all the years that had passed without my losing it. I had gone on the Scarsdale diet a few times, losing weight temporarily each time, but, the last couple of years—especially during the nine months of Teresa's pregnancy—I had gained it all back. I hit my old high of just over two hundred pounds, which I had first arrived at near the end of my time living in New York City.

It was the 1970s. I was leading, what I called at the time, an economically immature existence. I wasn't overweight at the start. I had published my first book in 1972, *The Harrisburg 7 and the New Catholic Left,* and lived in Milligan Place, a small courtyard enclave off Sixth Avenue between Tenth and Eleventh streets.

I was doing construction work in the South Bronx, at Feller's Scenery Studio. We built sets for Broadway shows. All the scenery traveled, and everything needed to fit into trucks. It was similar to doing house construction.

The job in the Bronx came from my contacts in the theater. During the summers I was in graduate school I worked for the Public Theater, Joseph Papp's organization. Feller's paid well and off the books (for the first year at least). I worked there two years, doing hard manual labor. And I ate like the laborer I was, large lunches of rice and beans at a Puerto Rican restaurant off the Grand Concourse and many cheeseburgers at the Cookie Bar on Hudson Street, which served the best burgers in the area, down a block from the better-known White Horse Tavern. I was very strong and not overweight. But finally I got a job that supposedly "fitted" my educational status.

Back then, a friend of mine, the lawyer Flo Kennedy, always gave me a hard time during my stints of working in the Bronx, for keeping some deserving less educated person from having a job. Feller's was a union shop, but he kept six miscellaneous laborers on staff, and the loyal brotherhood of the IATSE did not object, since nobody else wanted to do the work we did. During the six weeks my book was on the *New York Times Book Review*'s "New and Recommended" list, I was spending a lot of time in a garbage scow, out on the street next to Feller's building, dumping construction trash, making note of the fact that no other writers on the list (David Halberstam, Christopher Jenks, Margaret Truman, etc.) were sharing space with me. I knew I had made the wrong turn somewhere.

I started teaching in 1974, but I didn't change my eating habits (though the cuisine improved) and did little exercise, other than a lot of walking and fooling around with women. I gained weight; the muscle turned to fat. I was around two hundred pounds. I had a picture taken right before I left the city in 1978, standing in front of a Mack truck near my apartment on Charles Street, and I looked like the truck. Or at least a large fireplug.

‑‑‑‑‑‑‑‑‑‑

⟍⟍ In my hospital bed I came to the conclusion that Feller's almost killed me after all. (I thought it would be all the strange chemicals we were exposed to as we fiberglassed—Feller's was the first to use that material in set construction. We made Arthur Miller's *The Creation of the World and Other Business* out of fiberglass. It looked like a dozen Corvette bodies bolted together.)

My parents arrived at the hospital and visited briefly. I occasionally wonder what length a book of transcriptions of conversations between me and my parents would come to. More than this present volume? Less? There would be a lot of repetition in it (always a fear with any book, though) and not too many pages. Mostly, there would be a lot of meaningful silence.

My mother has had heart problems. She had a triple bypass in 1983. It is her side of the family that is riddled with atherosclerosis. All her siblings died of heart attacks. Her father had died young, and, lying in bed, I realized that that story was still somewhat unclear to me. He died unexpectedly, I knew that. It was a heart attack, I now was sure. My mother was barely a teenager.

I had a lot to find out, but it is certainly from her side of the family, though my father's mother also died of atherosclerosis—hardening of the arteries, as it was called then—in her late sixties (in addition she had what at the time was called dementia). My mother's parents weren't, like my father's, entirely Irish. Her father's last name was Kompare, and from my mother I had gathered he was "French," from Alsace-Lorraine. Perhaps his father or grandfather had been a deserter from Napoleon's army, hence the K in the name, instead of Compare, which would have looked French, at least. I had more or less believed that story for most of my younger days. A few years before my MI, it had become clear he was from some Balkan state. Slovenia, I think it finally became.[3] I used to joke that that's where my brains had come from, the Eastern European branch of the family. But ever since the former Yugoslavia broke up and the dominoes of nationalism started falling there, I no longer say it.

I was happy to see my parents. They were both subdued, especially my father, and if he is subdued, I know he is troubled. They left shortly after they arrived. I had been in bed for a couple of days, and it had been fourteen months, since Joe's birth, that I had gotten this much sleep. I was, though, not so much resting as recuperating. I was scheduled for an angiogram, where a radiopaque dye would be injected into my bloodstream and the heart and its arteries photographed. That would show what was what, I had been told.

An old acquaintance, Mark Kramer, nearly two decades earlier, had written a book on a couple of surgeons, following them around, observing operations, getting to know them. I had read it when it came out, first in *The Atlantic* and then as a book, called *Invasive Procedures,* which appeared in 1983. It was medicine as work. Such accounts seemed new at the time, a subset of the "New Journalism." Even the title: what surgeons did. Invade. So I had thought of any kind of surgery as just that.

Surgeons surge, I supposed. The procedure didn't seem to be much of an invasion and wouldn't be done by a surgeon but by a cardiologist. Thus far I had been invaded only by IV needles, most effectively by the "bolus" of tPA. This needle was to be a bit larger, and inserted through the thigh, hitching a ride on a large artery. I wondered why they didn't take that route for the tPA.

I was in the hospital's intensive care wing, the CCU (critical care unit), for four days, and then, the day before my cardiac catheterization, they planned to move me to another room, one in the PCU (post-critical care unit), with fewer machines, I presumed. For the last couple of days I had been musing on what was called my "minimal" heart damage. It had been a long time since I had been this inactive.

The last fifteen months had been the most difficult of my life. The sleep deprivation during the first six months of Joe's life had been crushing. Becoming a father for the first time at forty-four was, as we used to say in the sixties, a trip.

I had been a deep sleeper, and now, ever since Joe's birth, even when I could sleep for six hours at a stretch, it was a very light sleep, as if I were alert to any sound in the house, any intimation of danger. Lion with cub; it seemed to me something beyond culture.

But sleep was interrupted here, too. Someone would come in to check something, give me something. I would watch television, fall asleep, be awakened. After visiting hours the lights were dimmed. It was as if the hospital were flying across an ocean; the cabin lights were mainly extinguished, the staff moved quietly, picking up, moving on.

Among the medicines I was given each night was a sleeping pill. Not that my mind would be racing, but I had spent a lot of time watching the hills and valleys of the small green screen next to me, the heart rate numbers changing, going up and down by a few digits. It had been my exterior view into my interior, though I presumed the information was telling the doctors and nurses more than it was telling me. Since I was to be moved that evening, they hadn't brought me a sleeping pill, and, as the time went on, there weren't any preparations being taken to move me, either. I didn't much want to be asleep, then awakened to be moved, so I found myself getting agitated and upset, as it got later and later and I was neither asleep nor moved. The cardiac catheterization was to take place in the morning, and I wanted to be unconscious. I had spent too much time already contemplating the procedure and my condition.

I rang for the nurse, or, rather, pushed the button on the device that lay on my pillow. Eventually someone came, and I announced I wanted either the sleeping pill or to be moved now. She said that would happen soon, so I continued to wait. I continued to wait and stew.

⌐⌐ It was after midnight when they came to move me, and, because these folks were working the night shift, I'm sure it didn't seem like after midnight to them. More like the middle of their day.

But I started to complain, and though I was no longer getting any morphine, I was still able to hear myself. One part of me was mad; the other seemingly was listening to a guy feeling sorry for himself, making pronouncements, such as: All I wanted to do was to go to sleep four hours ago, and instead I've been up all night waiting to be moved, and tomorrow I'm having the most invasive procedure I've ever had. And look at my heart rate, I protested, pointing to the machine I was still hooked up to, at the numbers spinning Vegas-style up to the hundreds. Look at that! I said again, hearing the pathos in my voice, the voice of a stooge who doesn't get good service.

And so I was moved, rather silently. No one had much, or anything, to say to my complaints. I think they had all heard a variety of complaints and had seen a lot of folks who couldn't complain anymore, since this was intensive care, and not everyone was lucky enough to be moved to another room, other than the morgue.

Later that morning I was visited by a crisis manager from St. Joseph's Hospital human relations department. My venting the night before had been duly noted on my chart, and she was there to calm me down or soothe my nerves.[4] I suppose she was a true believer in free enterprise and thought I might be checking out of this particular Motel 6 and going to Memorial Hospital, only a few blocks away, but I didn't feel I was in a choosing position. No one from

Memorial had been making a pitch, and it had received some bad publicity a few years previously in the local paper for its very high mortality rates in just such matters of heart health management. It got the worse cases, was the hospital's argument, but people had been dropping like flies over there. Memorial had pledged to change its ways, according to the local paper.

The human relations woman was in the lovely person business, and she was indeed lovely. Memories of other people near death were never far away, given my circumstances, and I couldn't help recalling a good-looking social worker who visited my friend Inez (the woman I thought of as I walked with the old usher to the football stadium's first aid room) right before she slipped permanently into a coma. The social worker was supposed to talk to her about something delicate, sexual activity, or hygiene, or something. When she went in, I thought she must have gotten misinformation about Inez's extreme state. She came out very quickly and leaned against the wall, looking somewhat stricken, which I found oddly comforting, since it seemed so genuine. She was lovely—though one expected that in Massachusetts; there seemed to be such an abundance of healthy, vital, smart young women and men there.

Here, there wasn't an excess of attractiveness, but this woman's position required some. She told me the staff could tell that I would prefer a single room and that is why it took so long to move me. They knew one was coming vacant but weren't sure when that was going to happen, and they moved me to it as soon as possible, though she was sorry it turned out to be so late.

I pictured the "*I want a single room!*" vibes I must have been sending off for the past few days: One morose white male in his mid-forties who hasn't appeared very happy, or social, in his stay with us.

I recalled the time an older friend—Anthony Kerrigan, the Spanish translator and poet—had a heart attack, back in the mid-eighties. One night so many people were visiting Tony, it appeared that a New Year's Eve party had broken out. The crowd had finally been dispersed, and, in the middle of the night, before Tony was to have bypass surgery, he had another heart attack, which eliminated the reason to do the bypass. I had wondered why they couldn't have stopped that second one, though they had stopped his first, the one that had brought him to the hospital, with a shot not of tPA, but of streptokinase. I recalled his cardiologist describing Tony as "labial," meaning he loved to talk, and I certainly wasn't going to be so described.[5]

After the human relations woman left, I kept thinking of things I might have said to her. I hadn't said much, confirming everyone's psychological profile of me. Taciturn, etc. I should have said something like: My time here is going to be limited, finite, one way or another, so the fact that a large portion of it was made unpleasant is a big deal for me, if not for you.

But her purpose had been achieved. I wasn't completely mollified, but I had been attended to. Shortly after, I was prepped and wheeled away to have the cardiac catheterization.

The procedure wasn't very complicated, and it got them their pictures. A tube was inserted in my artery and made its way to my heart, and dye was expelled. The most acute feeling came when the dye flooded my heart. I felt my heart warm. It wasn't so much alarming as reassuring: I could feel it there, giving off heat.

I was mildly sedated and still in the aftershock period that follows an MI. The mind after such a blow often wants to bathe in the waters of amnesia, and, even though I resisted, the day or two after the attack remain the most cloudy. I remember thinking the machinery above my body sounded like a roller coaster clanking up the first incline as it was pushed into place to take the X-rays, which would reveal a nest of blood vessels and whether they were obstructed and by how much. But, of all the procedures, this one remained the least distinct. My hospital records were not too forthcoming, either. From the cardiac catheterization notes: "Left Heart Cath Via R Fem Artery, Findings, Pressures, Normal, Complications, None."[6]

I do recall lying still in bed for six hours with a "sandbag" over the wound on my upper right leg, the entry port, for hours. Since the vessel has been pierced, it needs the time to mend, to forestall complications. When I was finally able to urinate, I discharged a lot of tea-colored urine, which I presumed was the dye, filtered through my by now drug-abused kidneys.

Now they had proof, the cloudy X-ray images of my heart, the delicate fingers of veins that held it, clasped it, gave life to the muscle it was.

They had their map now and could describe the scene of the accident. Luckily for me, it wasn't in the "widow-maker" artery, the LAD (Left Artery Descending), but in the less important one, on the downside, the lower right portion of the heart, though my right artery was dominant. There it was: the site of the clot, now still cloudy, like a bruise. There were other plaque formations in my arteries, here, here, and there. Though nothing outstanding, the highest were 30 to 40 percent, most 10 percent, not figures that necessarily cheered me. What they wanted to do was an angioplasty—go in and push back the debris of the clot. That would had some salubrious effect, the doctor (the plumber of the cardiology group) said, though he didn't use the word "salubrious." It was just the thing to do.

Of course, he said, I could get another opinion, but if I didn't have it done, all that would occur was that I would probably fail a stress treadmill test before leaving the hospital and have bigger problems down the road. He said that brusquely, as if having a second opinion would be some sort of insult to him. He wanted to do the angioplasty. (Much later, I learned that cardiologists can do those procedures. That's where the money is. The even more lucrative bypass operations are performed by surgeons.)

"Down the road" was a problem for me at this point anyway. Would they make me take a stress test before I could leave the hospital? I liked the idea of something being done. It would have been odd just to leave the hospital without doing anything, other than having some chemical concoction eat through the blood clot. I'll ask around, I thought, see what the consensus is.

My class identity has always been mixed: part wage slave, part artist, academic, intellectual. My sister had married a doctor (a medical student at the time), though she was now recently divorced from him. Teresa's extended family includes doctors, so she made some phone calls. She found out that what was proposed was standard and that my "blockages" didn't appear to be major. I recalled something Dr. V. C. said to me before I was given the tPA: "You're surviving a heart attack, which means you have a 50 percent chance of surviving another one." At the time I thought my "surviving" was the 50/50 business, but I see now he meant "down the road." The next heart attack.

So the angioplasty was scheduled.

CHAPTER THREE

Infection

I had developed an infection at the site of the second set of IVs, the one done in the emergency room in my right hand. They had to get the infection under control before doing the angioplasty (or so I supposed), even though I had the infection when they did the ca-theterization. But I had been maintaining a fever, 101 degrees or so, and now it appeared to be something serious. They needed to find out exactly what sort of infection it was, to give me the specific an-tibiotic for it.[1] The infection appeared to be a resistant sort. This meant they needed to have a culture. Dr. V. C. was enlisted to get the specimen. He didn't seem afraid of infection himself, since I don't remember him wearing gloves.

It became your classic movie torture scene. I must have been cast in the role of the captured CIA agent, and he played a member of the intelligence force that wanted information from me. He kept pressing the wound, hoping to draw enough fluid to stain the glass plate. For some reason there wasn't an ample supply. I wasn't tied to the chair, but I had to pretend to be, to let him do what he wanted to do and not to pull away my hand.

This hurt; this was pain of the old-fashioned variety, not the heart attack's mystical state, or the vaulting experience of the tPA busting through the clot, the transforming reperfusion, as I discov-ered it was called—just regular pain. The doctor remained business-like throughout as he attempted to squeeze a few drops out, as if he were milking a rattler. Finally, he got what he wanted and left.

The angioplasty had been postponed until the infection was under control, but they hoped to reschedule it soon, in the next day or two.

After the "torture scene" I was brought a videotape on angioplasties to watch, so I would know what the procedure was like. They have videotapes on everything, I suppose. It turned out that the one they brought along wasn't on angioplasties, but since the equipment had all been set up, they showed it to me anyway. It turned out to be on phlebitis, which at least had something to do with veins and vessels and clots.

—⋀— I'm in bed, still recovering from the culture procedure, staring at the news on television. There are reports of Joseph Papp's death. I guess I knew he was suffering from some sort of cancer. As I mentioned in chapter 2, when I was in graduate school in New York City, I worked for Papp downtown at the Public Theater and for the Mobile Theater, which toured the city's boroughs. Papp's last wife, now widowed, lived in my former building, Milligan Place, before she married him. Nearly two decades later, in 1990, Papp and I had been on opposing sides (at least, early on) during the flap over the National Endowment for the Arts (NEA) controversies of the George H. W. Bush administration.

The controversy that swirled around the NEA was a legacy of the cash aesthetics of the Reagan years: it was a question not of truth and beauty, but what it's worth and who decides, a contest over value and control. Jesse Helms and the other conservative Republicans in Congress lusted for control; the idea of censorship was merely foreplay.

The "restriction" attached to the grants of 1990 only restricted what the NEA could do, not what individual artists could do. But the restriction was quickly turned into a "loyalty oath," a slanderous analogy, and that became the catchphrase. Artists were pitted against artists, as those who were opposed to the NEA wanted.[2]

Papp was for refusing grant money; I was for accepting and doing what one would with it. I was on the unpopular side, since any time you keep something, don't give something up, you don't appear to be a paragon of virtue. By the end of the controversy, Papp had turned down something like $750,000 of federal aid for his theater. Then, in early December 1990, he closed his scenery and prop shops and saved himself $750,000. The irony for me was extreme, given that was where I worked when he employed me. But I felt even more melancholy over his death as I lay in my hospital bed.

—⋀— The doctor who had been in the football stadium's first aid room dropped by to see how I was faring. I learned that he is a Notre Dame (ND) graduate and liked to volunteer his time at the stadium during football games. (And, in ND camaraderie, he came to visit.) He is an emergency room physician himself. He wanted to chat about Notre Dame, and the conversation quickly turned (or hadn't been anything but) social. I didn't ask him why he had been feeding me the hyperventilating baloney, but I had already con- cluded that since there wasn't much he could do, hyperventilating had been his placebo diagnosis, in order to get me to "relax," which seemed to be the ER physician's only mode of treatment until a car- diologist finally showed up.

The new antibiotic (Vancomycin) had gotten control over the hospital-supplied staph infection. The angioplasty finally was to take place. I had looked through the list of hospital services and saw that I could have my hair washed, so I scheduled that. I suppose I could have asked Teresa to wash my hair, but I thought of it as an equipment problem. I pictured a portable sink and other parapher- nalia.

It turned out to be just a young woman with a bowl and some shampoo—decidedly low tech. Having my hair washed before the angioplasty seemed important to me. It made me feel more hopeful, alive, fresh. Doubtless I was a bit musty. I hadn't had a shower since the day of my heart attack, some eight days earlier.

There was a beauty parlor on the first floor of the hospital, and she had come from there. I thought if Teresa had done it, it would have seemed too poignant. Having a stranger do it made it seem straightforward and efficient.

My parents and Teresa would be arriving soon for the big event. The idea of actual hardware being inserted into blood vessels and snaked up to the heart and made to expand all seemed on its face perilous. (Somehow, having a tube inserted into my artery and snaked up all the way to my heart didn't seem as invasive during the cardiac catheterization, since there was only dye to be delivered, not a mechanical event, an operation—the expanding of the artery—to take place.) But there was another peril. If, for some reason, anything went wrong, or the procedure provoked another heart attack, or couldn't be done, I would be whisked into the operating room and bypass surgery would be performed, if warranted. So it seemed not just an entirely discrete event (even though those outcomes were possible with just the catheterization). It might be just a prelude.

This wasn't a crack-of-dawn procedure, but took place in the early afternoon. I was transferred once again to a gurney and wheeled to a holding room. I was given ten milligrams of Valium. I hadn't much experience with drugs of that sort (or any pharmacological sort, though I had been given a sleeping pill, which must qualify), with anxiety reducers. My friend Robert badgered me into taking a Librium one evening back in the late sixties, and I finally did, while we were playing pool. It did seem to make the pool game rather stressless, and I shot well. It was decades later when they discovered that long ingestion of Librium was a risk factor for cervical cancer, which Inez, Robert's wife, died from.

I had hit upon my own way of distracting myself from the procedure while it was going on. I had read somewhere about "imaging," that it had some therapeutic effect. I couldn't recall on what (perhaps it was hitting a target with a bow and arrow, some Zen business: you imagine yourself doing it before you try to do it). So I was going to think of tunnels, of open tunnels, hallways, tubes; images of widening were to fill my head. That is what I had planned.

I was taken to some lower area of the hospital, to a room that did not look surgical. Rather, it looked like a place of manufacturing. It must have been the same place they did the catheterization. Everything seemed gray. The room was larger than it needed to be. It had frosty windows emitting a lot of gray light, and a glass-enclosed room down at one end. It reminded me of the day my wife and I had toured Bethlehem Steel.

We had walked through a rolling mill, along an upper catwalk, over a mile long. In one corner of the great hall was a glass-enclosed room, where men sat at computer consoles. They controlled the machinery, a mile of it, which reduced a thick slab of molten metal to a roll of thin coiled steel. On the rolling mill floor there had been only two men visible: one who walked along near the machinery that pinched the slab incrementally down, from a foot wide to less than a quarter of an inch, each roller reducing it further, and one man at the end of the process, who painted a serial number on the finished roll. When that man saw us up on the catwalk, he put a piece of paper towel on top of the roll of steel to show how hot it was. The paper towel burst into flames.

I was lifted inelegantly (I sagged in the middle) from one gurney to another and rolled into the room. I could feel myself smiling in a silly way (must be the Valium) and kissed my wife and my parents— what, goodbye? A short intense man came up to me and shook my hand heartily, introducing himself as the anesthesiologist, who was standing by, in case I needed to be hustled into surgery.

Even through the Valium I realized he was introducing himself, so when his bill arrived I would know who he was.

The color of medical equipment seems to be either a frothy seafoam green or an overcast gray. Around the operating table I lay on was an array of suspended machines, including a couple of television monitors. I could see off in the corner others in the small glass-enclosed room; that seemed to be a "control" room. My thigh was being prepared (they weren't going through the same holes the angiogram had used). I felt somewhat as if I were in the Navy, on a submarine. The round pipes holding wires and whatnot, along with heavier apparatus, were above and around me. I could momentarily see my heart, as the large disc-shaped image producer swung over my chest. The plumber doctor came in and said hello. He was the one who seemed to be insulted at the idea of my securing a second opinion. But since I didn't appear to have electrical problems, he now was going to be my primary cardiologist. I attempted to visualize all the tunnels, all the open spaces I could, to fill my mind with their images, once the team began its work. The insides of tunnels.

Something was being inserted into my artery, a long thin wire, a part of which had the capacity to expand. This I couldn't feel, though the cardiologist said I would feel "pressure" when the balloon operated. It was to reach the site of the lesion and expand, push the debris back against the wall of the artery. This was to have some positive effect, though I thought it might be better if the debris were eaten up, or flushed out, rather than just squeezed up against the walls, the interior of the poor, injured artery. But, I supposed, the more blood that flowed through the space, the more chance of it having some good effect, the power to heal.

So I thought of the Midtown and Holland tunnels in Manhattan, which went under the Hudson River to New Jersey. The white ceramic tiles gleaming in the headlights, the slightly flattened oval shape of the long tunnel, the rush of cars streaming through, the condensed roar of them all, the intensity of their size filling a small volume of space, at least in relation to the size of the cars and tunnels. Blood cells and arteries. How those white tiles gleamed! I recalled. How that tunnel held firm with all that water above it! I was in tunnel reverie. Then I thought of the one in Boston, and then various airports with their various tunnels leading to airplanes, all open, all clear.

The plumber doctor would occasionally yell out short words, as if he were communicating by voice alone with the folks in the corner room. The large wheel that took the pictures whirled about me, made a crescent sweep. It seemed like numbers, pressure readings, but finally I heard a whole sentence: "It's soft," he said.

I knew what "it" referred to: the site of the clot. His delicate machinery had reached the area and had begun to expand, inflate, push against the wall of the artery. This must be an important time, when the heart could stop again or, rather, another heart attack could be produced, since, while it inflated, the balloon too shut off the flow of blood. The numbers must be tolerances of allowable pressure. I expected to feel pressure, though what I felt was contraction, as if the artery was wrapping around the balloon, not the balloon pushing against it. I continued to think of open tunnels, gleaming white spaces.

It seemed that they were done. I thought I heard "withdrawing," some other words shouted out. The doctor abandoned his position by my side. The nurses in attendance began to fuss with me once again. Soon I was being wheeled out of the room, out from under the gray machinery.

My mother looked to be crying, my wife stared at me, and my father seemed his stoic self. The usual tableau: a family viewing a body in motion. It's a funereal image—the immobilized family, the coffin rolling by. I lost sight of them as I was pushed along.

Sandbags (of a white nylon variety) were put on my thigh, over the incision; they were to remain there for some hours, I was instructed. I was wheeled up again to the room I had left earlier.

It had seemed the procedure had gone well enough. I hadn't been hauled into surgery for a bypass. My heart did not stop; I did not have another heart attack, an MI. I did just have an angioplasty. I stopped thinking of tunnels, enclosed, elongated open space.[3]

CHAPTER FOUR
After the Catheterization

Once again, I lay abed with a sandbag on the wound. I had been through this before, after the angiogram, so it seemed simpler this time around. The wound is fairly large, the size of a ballpoint pen refill. Pressure needs to be maintained. Medicine is often primitive: they could have put a sandbag on a wound back in the Middle Ages. I began to wonder when sandbags were invented.

I was back in intensive care, or a post-op room, not the single room I was in before. I was to be released soon, I was told. But I had to be up and walking, and that would take a day or two.

The bag did not remain as long as the other did after the earlier procedure. Or I had become accustomed to it, and it didn't seem as long. I realized I had become adept at not moving much. There was no large volume of dye to expel. But there were plastic, strawlike sheaths to be removed. The wounds looked like the sort that would have been left by a very large rattlesnake bite.

I had spent an inordinate amount of time lying down. There was something quite fugitive about it. As if I were lying in wait, hiding, not wanting to be detected. I realized I was hiding from my body, keeping quiet so as not to disturb any of its sinister forces, as if the bad guys were around and they would get me if they knew I was here: real daydream sort of stuff. I listened for sounds, twinges, odd rumblings hitherto undetected. The body as minefield, ready to go off at any moment, triggered by one false step. It bred a physical paranoia that—I was surprised to discover—took months to lessen.

Visits and visitors were limited, except for Teresa. I thought of all those I had visited in hospitals. Usually their hospitalization was for something transient—or they were elderly.

I thought a lot about the birth of my son, a mere fifteen months earlier. Any near death experience tends to bring up its opposite, so I often thought back to the time before and after my son's birth.

My wife and I had done Lamaze classes, preparations for natural childbirth, at a different hospital, a part of a random group, bringing pillows, all with one condition in common: pregnancy. There were single mothers-to-be, with their mothers acting as support, and other nontraditional pairs.

We got to see a cross section of the community. One of the in-structors had brought along a child to demonstrate breast-feeding firsthand. She was behind a screen, and the instructors discour-aged—forbade, actually—the men from observing the actual dem-onstration. But she had discussed a few things at first and had used a doll for that purpose. She had been continually breast-feeding for at least five years, she reported. That seemed to be some extraor-dinary fact, but she was rather singular herself, which doubtless was why she was both a Lamaze teacher and a La Leche League volunteer.

She was comforting to look at, an embodiment of maternal beauty as cliché: bountiful, just a tad overweight, but well distrib-uted. The strangest thing about her, other than a life of constant suckling, was her eyes. I took very few drugs in the sixties, certainly none of the psychedelic sort, and the breast-feeding demonstrator had the most zapped eyes I had seen in a long, long time. If running can produce endorphins, she had tapped, through constant breast-feeding, some mother lode. I found her life unimaginable—and my wife thought it horrifying.

We had had strange visitors shortly after Joe was born. We were in the birthing section of the hospital, which appeared to be some sort of Motel 6. We had a view of the largely empty Uniroyal plant out the window. A dead fly sat on the sill. My wife had refused drugs, which an elderly nurse immediately offered her when we had arrived late the night before. She wasn't a regular birthing room nurse, but from down the hall, part of the regular delivery room staff.

But, finally, after a night of labor and an eventful but uneventful—as the doctors say—morning birth, all had calmed down following Joe's arrival. The three of us were lying on the bed, all in some shared daze, and two of my wife's graduate students arrived in the doorway. Hello, goodbye. They were the definition of inapropos, or, rather, seeing anyone at that moment seemed quite preposterous.

For the past few days, I hadn't had many visitors. Flowers and cards I got. But, as I lay in bed, I was still listening to my body tick, tick, trying to decide if there was any way to disarm it, to select what wire to cut, the red or green, before it went off again. I watched the machines, the rhythm of my heart, the rate of my pulse. I still had drips going. Television was on. And I was on the mend.

‿⋀‿ My wife's visits were not without reproach. Not on her part, but mine. I reproached myself. For many months before my heart attack Teresa would leave cut-out newspaper obituaries on the kitchen table of young men dead from heart attacks—most from the *New York Times* (that paper seemed to be a principal source, not so much our provincial local paper, where early death was usually the result of cars or gunplay, though the cause was often not mentioned.) But the *Times* was able to sample the largest pool of high achiever men in their forties and fifties kicking off.

I would look with mild exasperation at the clipping and read some version of the following: ". . . a chief financial officer of Coach Leatherware, died on Thursday at his home in Hillsdale, N.J. He was 39 years old. He died of a heart attack, a company spokeswoman said." Each clipping was a warning I chose not to take.

In 1983, I had driven to Chicago to attend the funeral for my Aunt Colette, who had died of a heart attack. My family was there, my mother having recovered from a triple-bypass operation she had two months before. My mother had lost weight, had stopped drinking, and seemed much younger, almost the way she had seemed to me when I lived at home in my late teens: she was sharp, somewhat acerbic. The absence of liquor made her testy; or, rather, there was no liquor to make her sentimental and remote.

My Aunt Colette, my mother's sister, was the most stylish of her siblings, a resident of the upscale Chicago suburb Glencoe, divorced when her children were teenagers. She had had a heart attack some eleven years before, in 1972. Because of my mother's attack and bypass operation, Colette had gone to her doctor for a checkup; she reported to my recuperating mother on the phone that she had received "a clean bill of health." Two weeks later Colette dropped dead of a heart attack while shopping at Marshall Field's.

At the funeral, in an open coffin, Colette's body was swollen— "with edema," my Uncle Joe said. He had spent a good bit of his adult life working as a tech in hospital laboratories.

It was then, at that suburban funeral parlor, that the cluster of deaths from heart attacks and heart troubles on my mother's side of the family finally began to loom large, too large to be ignored—or so one would have thought—despite the family's propensity to ignore them. My mother and her sister, one post-op, the other dead. Both my mother's two brothers still alive, but concerned. They were, as I was, adept at denial, however. It was then I began to hear a fuller version of my grandfather's death.

It wasn't from a plate in his skull, as I romantically remembered, the result of his fall from a balcony of the Iroquois Theatre, during a fire in 1903. And it wasn't from a heart attack. It was a cerebral hemorrhage, the result of bad genes, ailing arteries. But he did have a plate in his head and an angry red scar on his chest from the Iroquois Theatre fire, I learned.

My grandfather, Ralph Kompare, born in 1885, was one of Chicago's first Slovenian-American attorneys. His father ran a successful saloon. My grandfather arrived home from his office one day and found the triplex his family lived in on Coles Avenue under quarantine. Colette had contracted scarlet fever (her brother Jack had had it, and had been sent home too early from the hospital), and no one could enter. Ralph could talk through the front hallway door to his wife. He went to his office and stayed there for the week, but one night his brother saw the light on at night in the office, and he went in and found him dead on the floor outside the bathroom. It was 1934. Ralph was forty-nine.

My mother was eleven. There was no way of knowing if he had died immediately or had collapsed and lived for a while. But for a week he hadn't been able to see or touch or talk to his children, or to be with his wife.

Their financial circumstances changed. My mother's mother went into permanent mourning, and when my grandmother, whom we called Nanna, came into my life (or I came into hers), I knew her only as an eccentric woman, a widow forever, still in black, accentuated by long straight black (and gray) hair, with few comforts in her life, other than the Catholic Church. They had moved across the street, to the top apartment of another triplex, the cheapest one in the building, with slanted, oilcloth-covered walls. She babysat me often, so I have a number of memories of my times there. To me, she was always kind, but that didn't seem to be my mother's recollection. My grandmother could be cold and censorious, traits I undoubtedly share.

⎍ Melancholia certainly was my almost-daily visitor, as evidenced by my train of thought. If I had died, Joe would have no recollection of me, other than the most dim and buried. Most likely, he would have acquired one, through pictures, videos, and whatnot. He would remember me no more than I remember my mother's father, Ralph. But the thought of such things left me feeling weaker than I actually was. It was time to get up and walk around, so I could leave the hospital as soon as possible.

Near the end of my stay, I shuffled around by myself. Teresa had earlier taken me for a stroll down the hall, and, as I gripped the drip stand to roll along with me, I couldn't shake the notion of it being a staff, as if I were in darkness and some sort of light were dangling from the pole, not a plastic bag with solution in it, and I was to spend my days wandering, looking for myself, or an honest man. It was age that seemed to have descended on me. I was still forty-five, but a new kind of forty-five. I felt, wheeling the drip, shuffling along, transformed into an old man. Some clammy hand had touched me and left me weak.

Obviously, I had had a heart attack and two medical procedures in the last ten days, and I had been on my back in bed for most of the time, so I knew almost anyone would be weak after ten days in bed. The embarrassing hospital gown, the not-quite-a-shroud one wears, with little thin cloth ties holding it together in the back, added to the feeling of weakness.

So, not sleeping, I decided to take another walk around the floor—to start feeling more alive. There had been a new addition to St. Joseph's Hospital that I had observed driving by when it was being constructed. At that time, I wondered about the economics of it, the new wing that was being put on, since so much of it seemed to be only for show. The largest part was a new main entrance, with a tower of glass fronting the street, creating an atrium of sorts inside, a large empty space, seemingly without purpose, aping hotel construction, which, during the eighties, seemed to favor atriums.

The carpeting was still fairly new, the paint and woodwork all in muted taupe tones. I shuffled around, taking a slightly different route that led me to a small elevator, not one for patients, but visitors, a glass-enclosed cage, which traveled up and down within the new atrium entranceway. There was an open space, a balcony that ran some ten feet before a wall started again, and from the balcony I could look down and out over the open space.

Clinging to the silver rod of the drip stand, I started to tear up. The sight of the large empty space had an effect, the glass wall on the other side revealing the parking lot, the street beyond, the one I had driven down so many times as all this was being built. I'm not sure if it was the "beauty" that was making me emotional, the sight of captured space and the inherent wonder of it, the sense of expanding possibility it embodies, the beyond, the future, the vista of all that remains, but it truly had an effect. Just the enclosed space provoked a response.

This is why they built it, I said to myself, so some wretch like me could be moved by it, to have some emotional experience on a walk

around the corridors, to counter the oppression of the claustropho-
bia that comes from being in a hospital room. It seemed generous,
something I had not been when I used to assess the why and where-
fore of its construction. I had thought it was for show.

And it was for show. To show me. Something. I shuffled back to
my room. There was mainly silence. A few nurses were in their central corral, behind a short wall, working at desks and computers, filling out forms. I passed the patients' small rooms, the stub ends of
beds visible, chairs, a muted disquietude most often within. Those
people I saw were old, elderly. I appeared to be the youngest person
in the neighborhood.

I was alone, and it seemed to me that I had been alone a lot the
last ten days, though Teresa, when she had visited earlier, had said
something that had puzzled me. She said she liked the fact we got to
talk so much. She, I supposed, was looking for silver linings. The
amount of talking we did didn't seem much out of the ordinary to
me, though the circumstances were certainly not ordinary. It seemed
like the same sort of conversation we always had. We had been
married since 1986. We had eloped. Since I was forty at the time and
it was my first marriage, I definitely wasn't the marrying kind. My
life had taken a variety of turns, and getting married was a big one
for me.

⎯⋀⎯ Though it was now becoming clear that the atherosclerosis
came flowing down the genetic river of my mother's side of the family, I felt compelled to look at my father's side, too. His mother
died of "hardening of the arteries," as it used to be known. I had her
death certificate—for a curious reason: I had obtained a copy of it
from my family way back in 1969, when I was unsure of what I
wanted to do about the draft. One option was to become an Irish
citizen, since one needed only one Irish-born grandparent to qualify.
My grandmother's death certificate provided that proof.

My father's father lived to what used to be called a ripe old age.
After my grandmother, his first wife, died, a few years passed, and
he hitched up with a Jewish widow (at least I always assumed she
was Jewish), Mabel, and married her. That's where the family for-

tune went—to Mabel. I think it consisted of about three shares of stock in the Illinois Central Railroad, his former employer. My father, it appeared, had inherited his longevity.

But it was my father's father who was the only one of his brothers to get married, and it was his father, my great-grandfather O'Rourke, who had been the immigrant from Ireland at the end of the nineteenth century and had finally noticed that none of his sons were married, or seemed to have much interest in matrimony. My great-grandfather's sister went back to Ireland for a visit, to County Mayo, and an acquaintance asked her if she knew of a boy who might be interested in his daughter, who was planning to immigrate. She said she knew of four. It was Bill, my grandfather, the most malleable of the bachelor sons, who eventually wed her. That's how my grandmother, Ann Clark, was procured. She almost didn't make it over to the New Country, since she had passage booked on the *Titanic*, but, nearing departure, she had changed the ticket in order to travel with another village girl who was also going to America but couldn't leave for a few weeks.

Every lineage can look backwards to some moment when extinction was avoided, and that's one of ours.

But not being married at forty seemed to be handed down, just as certainly as the plaque lining my arteries was handed down DNA to DNA, and I began to contemplate what that emotional mix added to the stew of my thick blood. I had always been proud that I coagulated so quickly when cut. Now I realized that that "sticky" blood wasn't the boon I thought it to be.

My wife wasn't sent for from County Mayo, but arrived fresh from graduate school at the University of California, Berkeley, to a job in the Notre Dame economics department. I had come to Notre Dame at the start of the Reagan era, tracking the Gipper's footsteps. I always thought I had my finger on the pulse of my generation, so I thought it was somehow fitting—leaving the East Coast and returning to the Midwest, something I never thought I would willingly do. I had grown tired of being a gypsy writer, going from school to school on short term contracts, subsidizing my writing of fiction. As they say, I hadn't had a "breakthrough" book, one that put me into the popular culture orbit, where one can make a living at writing.

Like so many of my generation, I was teaching writing. Notre Dame made the best offer the year I looked only for tenure-track jobs, and so here I was in a dying Midwestern industrial small town.

So Teresa's arrival was welcome indeed. She seemed to be both a link back to my old life (her counter-culture Berkeley aspect, being an educated woman with progressive ideas) and a bridge to a new one (she is eleven years younger than I). I had never been to the West Coast till I met her, having always gone no further than New Mexico in my past, but here was the old admonition, "Go West, young man," writ large for me, a fresh start for what I hoped would be the second half of my life.

We got married in Las Vegas, at the most tasteful of all the wedding chapels, the Little Church of the West, in early July, in between the marriage of her cousin to Teresa's boss's son and the marriage of my youngest sister to her boss's son. Since both of those weddings had been planned for over a year, I didn't feel bad about eloping (we kept it a secret at the time, but, since we didn't remove our rings when we attended the second wedding, my sister Amy's, it came out then). And Teresa had been married before, absolving me, I told myself, of the need to provide a large, public ceremony for her. (Not that that was in any way the correct assumption.) What we had was the first marriage of the day in a little chapel, something that looked dollhouse-like, set off by itself on the strip near the Hacienda hotel and casino.

Our witness (the chapel's manager) swept the front walk during the ceremony, and some Australian tourists who drove up as we were leaving took some snapshots for us. I had won the price of the ceremony at Caesar's Palace the night before at blackjack. We were happy. And we went back to the Vagabond Inn to pack and go swimming, and Teresa dove into the blue pool wearing her contact lenses, and I spent some time locating and fishing them out, two darker blue dots floating in the sparkling water.

We went to the Grand Canyon for our one-day honeymoon and stayed at the El Tovar, the old Teddy Roosevelt–era hotel on the South Rim. We were driving a repossessed car (having flown to Sacramento for the first wedding, we needed a way to drive to Vegas and beyond), which needed to be delivered to Phoenix, Arizona, where an old friend of mine was a film critic for the *Arizona Republic*. Though I didn't tell her the purpose of the trip, she divined it, since Las Vegas was the central point, and she threw us a small wedding party when we arrived, mid afternoon, when it was 114 degrees, after dropping off the car at the bank that wanted it back. We flew on the next day to my sister's wedding in Kansas City.

Those did seem the carefree days, but the last years seemed far less carefree, indeed. The last two had been especially hard. Teresa had a couple of miscarriages before Joe was conceived. One required a D & C (dilation and curettage), after progressing a few weeks. The ultrasound showed a dark, still mass. She seemed to become frantic with the need to be pregnant.

Even though she had to be pregnant to have miscarriages, she felt I should go to a doctor to be checked, so my sperm could be evaluated, and I wondered what had happened to us, since everything now appeared to be a question of utility.

But she did become pregnant fairly quickly again. And this time, for all nine months, I thought myself—and was—a nervous wreck, while Teresa was thoroughly and healthily pregnant. I was never more anxious than during those months. Finally, Joe was born.

Thereafter, I was introduced to clinical sleep deprivation, the boot-camp period of having a first child.

The last two years before my heart attack had been harder and harder still, since my career had become thoroughly becalmed. I had felt plateaued out, as they once described the phenomenon in the music business.

The novel I was writing about the English coal miners, *Notts,* didn't appear to be a breakthrough book in the making. I had put on weight; my exercise was limited. I had a little boy, and I hadn't realized that just keeping him alive would be such a difficult matter and that fatherhood would be such a powerful producer of so much vigilance and anxiety.

So I stared at the board on the wall in the hospital room with my weight and height, the weight being, I thought, too high, and the height being too short.

Both sides of my family tree, it now seemed clear, had conspired against me. I found myself wondering, for the first time ever, whatever became of my grandfather's brothers, the ones who never married, never had children. I couldn't remember ever meeting them. They, childless and wifeless, had been lost to history, or at least to mine.

⌁ Ten days after I entered the hospital I was to be released.[1] One night I saw a doctor from the cardiology group (that claimed my share of Blue Cross coverage) making rounds. I asked him if there were any restrictions on sexual activity. He looked at me quizzically and said, "Oh, what is it? They say having sex uses up as much energy as walking up a flight of stairs. I'd be careful for a while. Let her do most of the work."

He departed. I recalled when Tony Kerrigan, my now dead friend (of cancer, not the heart attack he had earlier), claimed that while he was in the hospital when the prostate trouble was first found, he had sex with his girlfriend, some five decades his junior, who was, for a while, to become his co-wife, during a period of temporary bigamy that Tony had arranged. (It's a long story. His *New York Times* obituary is a monument to the confusion.) He also said that a nurse had discovered them and was aghast.

I was trying to sort out at what: the medical consequences, or the age difference, or just the libidinous activity, but Tony gave me to believe it was more oral sex than anything quite as demonstrative as full pelvic contact.

With the sleep deprivation of the last fourteen months, nightly feedings, etc., the sex was not all that frequent anyhow, but I wanted to know. It was the pervasive weakness, enforced by lying down, that I wanted countered.

The doctor who did the angioplasty came by shortly before I left, since it was his signature that would release me. (I was to see my new internist a week or so after I got out of the hospital.) My angioplasty doctor wrote prescriptions for nitroglycerin and Cardizem, and, on his way out the door, I asked him about cholesterol-lowering drugs I had been reading and hearing about.

"Oh, is your cholesterol high? I'll give you another," and he wrote a prescription for Mevacor. By this time, I wasn't surprised by such cavalier dispensing of drugs.

I would be checking into his office for cardio-rehab and examinations, in any case, next week.

There was a flurry of papers to be signed, instructions given by nurses; I still needed to watch out for the angioplasty entry wounds and should restrict myself to very limited activity. I would be seeing a nutritionist at cardio-rehab (which I supposed would eliminate the bad pork chops). Teresa still couldn't believe that they served me pork chops. *A* pork chop, I assured her.

Though I had been shuffling around, I wasn't allowed to walk out of the hospital but was helped into a wheelchair, which a nurse rolled, my wife alongside. We brought home some of the plants that had been sent during my stay.

It was a sunny day, early November, a slight winter chill, and I realized it was the first time I had been outside in a long time. In fact, I had never *not* been outside for ten days at a stretch before in my life.

The blue sky began to occlude, as if the gray winter tones were asserting themselves. The light was tempered. Winter was on its way.

I was warned again about too much jostling of my leg. I was not to drive for a few days. I managed to get into the car's front seat, reclined, so I could stretch out the leg. My wife was driving, something that had always been a source of conflict, my liking to drive and not sharing it 50/50, as she wished to, as we were sharing the looking after of our son. Though, for the last ten days, I hadn't been sharing any looking after.

I was still to recuperate at home, in bed. It was cost-saving to get me out of the hospital room. I remembered our return to our house with Joe, after being in the other hospital not even twenty-four hours, always awake. We began Joe's life sleepless and hadn't yet caught up.

Carrying him to the front door had been a preternatural experience. Doubtless from the lack of sleep, but also from the effect of his birth. Everything to me appeared covered with radiance, aura, shine.

This time the return wasn't as glowing. The sky had turned gray. I thought of the day I rushed out of the house to my car on the way to the football game—where was the car!? There, parked across the street. My wife had brought it back during the week.

I hobbled up to the front door, and my father opened it, and I walked into the hallway. My mother stood behind my son, who was standing looking at me, an expression of worry on his face. I picked him up in my arms, with what felt like a surge of strength, and hugged him.

"Hi, Joe. Boy, am I glad to see you."

Teresa was behind me carrying plants. My father went out to car to help gather the other things.

I put Joe down. He still looked wary, concerned. I looked around. I had missed Halloween, I saw from the decorations, the carved jack-o'-lantern. Otherwise, the house looked the same, but it was never to be the same again.

CHAPTER FIVE

A Shadow Biography

In any life there is a shadow biography, a life with medicine and contact with doctors. One can pick a strand of anything to chart a life: what one wears, for instance. How that changes, what it says about you, the economy, society in general. Having a heart attack makes this sort of reviewing unavoidable. You revisit them all, more or less, one at a time, for the question that gnaws at you is: Could my heart attack have been prevented?

I was born in a car, or so I believed for a while. Some sort of accident on the way to the hospital. But that wasn't entirely the case. My mother got to a hospital, though there was some sort of car trouble along the way.

I had my tonsils out when I was five or six. It was the beginning of the fifties, when they were taking practically any kid's tonsils out. If one child had them out, why not a sibling? My generation was cut without much thought: circumcision was run of the mill; tonsils being snipped was equally pervasive.

But I remember the trip, before dawn, from our house to the hospital, entranced by the dashboard glowing in the disintegrating darkness. My parents were both sweet to me, which I enjoyed, though, since I was to be operated on, they were probably feeling sentimental.

The anesthesiologist said he would give me a penny for every number I could count as I received the gas, and I think I got up to twenty-three. I had also been promised ice cream to eat, which sounded like a treat, after the operation. I awoke in an old iron bed, which had been covered with thick white paint, in the children's ward. There were many beds, but most were unoccupied. I threw up dark red, heavy blood into two shiny, stainless steel, kidney-shaped bowls. Then I got my ice cream.

I got my pennies and was given my tonsils and adenoids, too, in a small brown bottle, which I kept till I was about twelve; by then the formaldehyde evaporated and the contents dried up, into bean-like shapes, and I finally threw the bottle away.

I was taken to the emergency room a couple of years after the tonsillectomy. An older girl offered to take me for a ride on her bicycle, down a steep hill near our house. I think I was sitting on the handlebars or the front fender, and she got going so fast she lost control, and we took a spill at the bottom of the hill. I ended up with a bump on my head and may have been unconscious for a moment. My mother came running after a girl had gone to the house and said I was dead. I was examined at the hospital but pronounced undamaged, other than the bump, and my mother took me and my older sister to a hamburger drive-in. I remember the afternoon and the event as sun-struck and sleepy, though the trip to the drive-in seemed both magical and warm, another unexpected treat, like the ice cream.

A couple of years after that, I was back in another emergency room. I had fallen off a three-step ladder jumping into a wading pool in our backyard. I fell onto the hinge of the ladder as it started to fold up and cut a horseshoe-shaped gash in my leg. I could see through to a large blood vessel, happily unsevered, and there wasn't much blood from the torn flesh itself. Thinking I shouldn't put much stress on such a fragile-looking thing as that crimson tube, I crawled to our back door and up the stairs and was taken to the hospital, with a towel wrapped around the wound.

As I was wheeled into the operating room, a nurse said, Oh, the doctor's so good, you won't even have a scar.

I, of course, have a large scar, a pronounced horseshoe branded onto the back of my leg, behind the knee.

There were dentists in between these occurrences. The same family dentist all my childhood. Nothing dramatic happened there; except at one point, braces were mentioned, since one of my front teeth protruded a bit. But I was playing grammar school football, and a boy charged into my helmet first and drove the tooth back straight. Regular checkups and only a few cavities.

Also around the cavity time, as a teenager I went to a doctor to get a checkup for a school form, and he asked me how long it had been since I had done anything for my skin. For some reason, I thought he asked how long I had been a thespian. I had acted in high school plays, something, however improbable, he could know. And I had bad skin. I realized I had misheard, and after saying, sprightly, a couple of years, I answered his original question without his asking it again. I hadn't done anything, except for making use of the world of over-the-counter acne products.

He seemed angry I hadn't had professional help. I told my parents, and they made an appointment with a dermatologist who was treating a friend's daughter. That was my first experience with any long-term care, an ongoing condition. I was a high school senior.

My parents were making a typical American journey in the late fifties, early sixties. They were moving from the lower middle class to the middle class. My father's father worked all his life for the Illinois Central Railroad, despite being an alcoholic for most of it. My father, during World War II, worked for the Pullman company building airplanes. He had enlisted in the army at the beginning of the war, but at that point they were being more selective than later, and his vision washed him out. Later, when he might have been accepted, he didn't attempt to enlist again. The Pullman work was good. After that he got the job that he kept all his life, working for a small bearing company that was eventually, at the end of his career, bought by a large company, and he was more or less phased out.

But going to the doctor was always seen as an exception, a last resort. So when the idea of my going to a dermatologist was raised, he said, "Oh, everyone has zits," but since my mother wanted me to go, I went.

This was in the very early sixties, and the doctor I was sent to, by chance, used X-ray treatments. I was happy enough with the idea that my complexion could be made better, so I, like my parents, went along easily, no matter how weird it all seemed at the time. My eyes would be covered with lozenges of lead. Thick rubber would be laid over the part of my skull containing my brain, and a bulky X-ray machine would be turned on, after the nurse had left the room and secured the door. She looked through some safety-glass window, and every once in a while during a treatment she would stop it and adjust the slab of rubber that had slipped off my head.

The doctor, after the first visit, didn't administer the treatments, and I would see him only once in awhile disappearing into another room filled with blue light, wearing what looked like welding goggles. But I went through the course of treatments, which spanned a little over a year, and after a while finally got to see the doctor again and wondered about their efficacy. He said, unhappily, "Well, you were hopelessly scarred when you came and now you are improved." He seemed displeased I had questioned his judgment.

Other than that, I was a healthy enough teenager and young man, but as the years went on the memory of those treatments grew more alarming whenever I would see any history of medicine looking back on the "bad old days." The contraptions in the photographs were all too reminiscent of the X-ray and the lead eye coverings and stiff slabs of rubber. One, of course, wonders about what used today will look equally alarming decades from now.

Throughout college and graduate school I hardly ever saw a doctor professionally.

I knew a psychiatrist socially; his wife had been my teacher. And another shrink had written me a letter that helped me evade the draft during the Vietnam War. His name had been provided as someone sympathetic to draft resistance. This was 1969. For a number of years, the early sixties, I had been a premature anti–Vietnam War protestor. I had been thinking of going to jail (as I saw it—though I might have ended up going to court, dragging it out for years), or letting myself be drafted, or getting out. In the end I chose getting out.

While finishing graduate school and living in New York City, I had a job, though so low paying I was able to use a government program that allowed me to have a physical for a dollar at a downtown New York hospital, one of the largest. I decided to have one, since I was about to leave town. It was a brief period (late sixties, early seventies) of wonderful social services for the poor.

When I showed up for my appointment, I had a long wait, but was finally called in and met an older Jewish physician, somewhere in his sixties. He looked at me and said, What are you doing here?

I said I had come for a physical. I had had a swollen gland, at least I thought it was a gland, high up on the inside of my thigh, and that was what made me think of getting a physical, but by the time I had gotten an appointment, the swelling had disappeared.

But I told him about it, and he looked at me skeptically. Then he said he wanted to conduct the interview in French, since he was tired of speaking so much Spanish, as he had been doing to the long line of people he had been seeing. I had told him I just got out of graduate school, and he took it for granted I could speak French, which I really couldn't, but I could stumble my way around in it in tourist fashion, which I did.

After he looked me over, he dropped the French and asked how many beers did I, as a good Irishman, drink a day? I told him some conservative number, and he said I probably should drink less and perhaps I should have my skin looked at; there were specialists in the hospital who could offer some treatments. I told him of the early teenage X-rays, and he examined my thyroid gland again, since that's where most of those treatments ended up causing damage. He said they don't do that sort of thing anymore. But the hospital's doctors probably could do something beneficial.

He sent me away to take some lab tests, which I took, but I couldn't make an appointment with the dermatology department early enough to find me still in town, so all that got postponed to life down the road. He was a pleasant guy who had shown some interest, though I didn't see another doctor for nearly five years, this time in the Florida Keys.

I was there with a girlfriend visiting friends and developed some sort of rash on my penis, which I had found annoying enough to have checked. I was on Sugarloaf Key, staying with Robert and Inez, and the doctor had an office in his house not too far away.

This was late 1974, and when I told his nurse/receptionist what I wanted looked at, she said, Uh oh, and when he came into the examining room, he said, Have you been using that much? And I said, yeah, I guess, and he just thought it was a friction burn, or that some coral dust had irritated it, or something, but it wasn't anything to be concerned about. He said for treatment I should just give it a rest and read a book.

I had, by then, developed the theory that men often get examined indirectly, since women went to doctors so often. Ricochet treatment. For a while, during the late seventies, I even dated a medical journalist, so I thought I was being kept abreast of the latest information. Examinations by osmosis. I still have the original, stapled-together-on-brown-paper version of *Our Bodies, Our Selves.*

Of course, economics had a lot to do with it. When I finally got a teaching job and joined the ranks of the regularly employed, I did go to doctors. I had developed small skin flaps, tags, I think they are called, in the area of my armpit and saw a dermatologist on Cape Cod. He removed them, saying they were harmless, some people get them, some don't, but when he discovered I was a writer, he wanted information on summer writing workshops, since he was thinking of attending one.

I took false pride in never having had a "social disease" (all that good medical care the women I knew were getting), but finally I might have acquired one, though there weren't any symptoms. My medical journalist had come down with trichomoniasis, and I got a phone call from her doctor saying I should take a remedy (Flagyl) just in case, which he would prescribe over the phone. What pharmacy did I use? The picturesque one on Sixth Avenue.

I then told another woman I had been seeing concurrently, in case this was being passed around, even though I might not be infected. She didn't take that news particularly well, especially when I learned later she had gotten a prescription filled (she evidently had the malady before), and no one informed her she should not drink alcohol while taking the medication, and she did, which made her feel awful.

This was the 1970s in New York City, if that is, in any way, explanatory.

I left the city to teach at Mount Holyoke College in Massachusetts in 1978. It appears, from all evidence, that I left the city right before the AIDS epidemic began. I've wondered, given the number of women I knew in the city as a single man, what would have occurred if I had stayed in New York through the eighties. I must admit, though, I left town because my glorious life with women was slowing down or, much to my surprise, becoming more work than I had imagined or wished for.

Since my first academic job in 1974 I had had health insurance, but that didn't send me to doctors for checkups, or the like. Just, as I have discussed, when the occasion arose.

But, in an highly ironic way, I was very much a man alone when I taught at Mount Holyoke, surrounded by hundreds of young women. For some reason, I didn't believe one should date students, though that certainly didn't impede many of my colleagues.

I wrote a long lovelorn novel, entitled *Idle Hands,* during the three years I was there, and that had something to do with it. I was busy, though I did become briefly involved with a couple of faculty women.

A man alone doesn't have much incentive to take care of himself. It was 1978, and the jogging and fitness craze had just taken hold. I did attempt a little running, but that doesn't do a whole lot unless it is accompanied by calorie deprivation, and I wasn't depriving myself of food.

That is when the weight really settled in, since my physical activity was limited. Three years of Stouffer's TV dinners and the like, long before the fast food industry became fat conscious. I seemed to have the same consciousness as the mass media does; when it turned, I was ready to turn, but not until.

One of the perks for the Mount Holyoke faculty was the chance to have free instruction at a two-week summer tennis camp, which

I took advantage of my second summer there. One of the things they do to justify the large fees that the out-of-towners paid was videotape the campers practicing. I watched my tape and wondered, Who is that tree trunk shuffling over the court? My backhand improved, but I still didn't lose much weight. But I would say, I know I should lose some weight.

My lovelorn novel came out just before I left Mount Holyoke, and I gave a reading from it. Some of the posters for it were defaced: THIS BOOK INSULTS WOMEN. But the reading was well attended, and the poster critics hadn't actually read the book, so the crowd didn't tear and rend me. I did run into Maxine Kumin, the poet, whom I hadn't seen in a number of years, and she looked at me rather alarmed. "Bill, you've gotten so big." She has a motherly streak, which is a side of women I hadn't seemed to tap much over the past decade.

I had become involved with a woman who did run; she was from an upper-middle-class Baltimore family, and, other than drinking a lot, she was fairly health conscious. I did discover some pressing need at her mother's home, where we were visiting. I left a day before I was scheduled to, because I was having what amounted to an asthma attack. It was some high form of allergy that her mother's house brought on: feathered pillows, dust mites, cats, orchids? Probably all, but it was bad. By the time I had acknowledged it (I had been toughing it out) and finally was advised to get an over-the-counter remedy, the nearest drugstore was just about to close. But the mother patronized it, a venerable old apothecary, and even though I arrived five minutes past closing, they let me in, and I bought an inhaler.

That helped. But I took off that night for the Cape, where I would be joined by my friend after concluding her visit with her mom. I had been suffering, as they say, from allergies for many years, but I had thought it just ordinary fact that one's eyes and nose would run for months at a time. One thing about distilling from one's life, only one aspect—in this case the medical—and tracing it along a lifeline is that it certainly exposes one as a mess. (And, God forbid, self-absorbed.) I didn't, at the time, seem quite such a mess as I am describing. I just put up with a lot; that was how I looked at it.

My Baltimore friend and I became my first thoroughly domestic union. I had never actually lived with a woman. Manhattan never made that necessary. People often kept two apartments even if they eventually got married in the city. Such was the hold of real estate over romance in the 1970s.

I left the East Coast for the Midwest, and we found a rented farmhouse amid soybean fields, corn, and pig farms. It didn't take me long to look for an allergist. All one needed was a phone book. This was still before managed care, but BlueCross BlueShield had some relationship with the local clinic, so I went there.

My allergist was always on the verge of treating my high blood pressure, but he remained only on the verge.

My friend from Baltimore and I parted more amicably than one might imagine, since I was the cause for her moving to this part of the Midwest. But I didn't feel all that culpable, because she had left a job in another part of the Midwest for a better one in the same region that allowed us to set up housekeeping. Had I dragged her here from the East Coast, I might have felt more guilty.

Nonetheless, I found myself alone, and I abandoned farm life for the not-so-big city. Then I met Teresa, my first "younger woman," younger than I, at least. Since I had finally lived with one woman, it wasn't too difficult to have another move in, though Teresa moved in to stay. My allergies were under control, and Teresa too was a runner, but seemed eminently healthy because of her relative youth. Being from California she brought with her a more up-to-date notion of healthy living.

During that period (circa 1984), on and off I would, after a cold or flu lingered for more than ten days, take myself to a Doc in the Box to be checked and to score some antibiotics. I would tell the doctor about my green phlegm and nose mucous, and I would be looked at and have, among other things, my blood pressure taken. It would be high.

One doctor suggested I have my blood pressure checked with some regularity. He said the readings could go up and down quite a bit, but if I had a series of readings it should be more or less accurate. I had heard of the white coat syndrome, in which doctor visits alone drove up blood pressure readings. My internist and I had talked about that in the past. A colleague of mine at school took his own blood pressure readings. And there were machines at the local drugstores, where you sat down and a blood pressure cuff tightened over your arm and a digital reading came forth. I had done that a number of times. I was always at the high end of the borderline reading. Those contraptions reminded me of the shoe-store machines of my youth, where you would look down at your feet through a crude eyepiece and see, thanks to an emitting X-ray machine, the green glow of your feet through your shoes. All this just to see if you had enough room to wiggle your toes. Those devices had finally been taken out of the stores, a bit before my bouts of X-ray treatments had been begun by the dermatologist.

The Doc in the Box gave me a card and said there would be no charge for checking my blood pressure. Just come in and get a reading. I'm not one to turn down a bargain (shades of my dollar charge for that New York hospital checkup long ago). I still have the card, pressed soft and frayed at the edges. The readings are even more alarming now than they were then. On January 23, 1989, the first visit with my cold symptoms, my left arm was 152 over 112; my right arm was 160 over 128.

I went back two days later, feeling a bit better. The reading was 152 over 110 in my right arm. A different doctor was there that day, and he said, with emphasis, that I better do something about that blood pressure, because with it I could certainly have a stroke. I told him I had just come from exercising (which I had), and he said, alarmed, "Exercise is supposed to lower your blood pressure, not raise it."

I went back on February 15, 1989, and it was (left arm) 158 over 108. I'm sure I was somewhat concerned; I cut back on the number of Doritos, all the salty snacks I had been eating, and went back on February 27. The right arm was 142 over 90. In two weeks, I went again, and the readings were 120 over 102 in the right and 130 over 92 in the left. Then on March 17, I went, and they were 130 over 98 on the right and 120 over 92 on the left. Those were close to what I had been getting on the drugstore machines, so I stopped checking at the Doc in the Box, having been lulled by the decrease in the numbers.[1]

I told the dermatologist I had been seeing once or twice a year about my tendency to high blood pressure, and he said I looked healthy to him. (I'm still not sure what prompted that remark, since I had been going to him because my skin was unhealthy.) Before the Doc in the Boxes opened, I had gone to a different physician who was taking walk-ins with my usual bad cold, and he said he was going to make me feel better, which I took in a hopeful manner, though he was also reassuring about my blood pressure, which had been high, but not that high that day.

It was obvious even to me that I belonged to the glass-half-full school of thought where it concerned my blood pressure. Diet could lower it, though, at best, to the high end of borderline high. If a doctor had said to me, "You must take medicine," I wouldn't have objected. I just didn't try to prompt anyone to tell me that.

During the summer before the heart attack, I had developed a sore on my index finger. The sore became a large infection, a pustule of a sort that looked like it needed to be lanced. I had been expecting it just to go away or to drain itself, but the skin seemed tough around it, and it was annoying me every time I reached into my pocket.

So I took myself again to a Doc in the Box (it was a Saturday afternoon after a wedding reception when I finally got fed up with it). The doctor there gave me a shot of Novocaine and lanced it as I looked away. Earlier, the nurse had taken my blood pressure, which was—surprise!—high.

When the site of the IV became infected, I told the doctor about that sore I had had a couple of months before. He seemed reassured, as if that explained the infection at the site. I suppose it made it seem less likely it had been a hospital-acquired infection (though that is what it appeared to be).

During the year before the heart attack, I had a series of night sweats. It was amazing how wet the sheets had become. I thought I was fighting a fever. But, in retrospect, they seem much more ominous. They ran for a period of a few weeks, then ceased.

After a heart attack one can't help reassessing one's earlier medical care. Mine was so-so and slap dash. My allergies were better. My skin was still troubled. Heart attacks are often called a lifestyle disease, only because cancer and other diseases aren't thought to be directly acquired through one's choices in diet and exercise. But life-style eventually laps over onto other diseases, cancer-related smoking, for instance. There are those who think living under power lines or too close to nuclear generating stations, or polluted water or air, contribute or play a role in etiology. Environmental sources are often the subject of litigation.

My brushes with various doctors and cardiologists over the last decade have left me with the equivocal position that half of them think problems such as mine are genetically predisposed and life-style has little to do with it; the other half think lifestyle does play a major role. I go on the assumption that it is both, though genetics might be leading my parade, since my culturally acquired liking for certain diets of death may be themselves linked to genetics in some fashion or another.

The question ("Could my heart attack have been prevented?") remains somewhat unanswerable. But I'm inclined to believe that if my untreated high blood pressure had been treated, my heart attack might have been prevented. The question remains: Would I have changed the way I ate and altered my penchant for no exercise if I had not had a heart attack?

In other words, was the heart attack good for me?

I cringe to admit it, but I do recall during the year before my heart attack wondering if the best thing would be to have one and survive it. I would have not wanted to think such a thing, but my memory is that I did think it once or twice before I actually had the attack. From your mouth to God's ear, etc.

CHAPTER SIX

The Lucky Disease

Heart attacks are the lucky disease. "Aren't you lucky," I heard quite a bit, in a variety of forms, after I left the hospital. Then I would be told different reasons for my good fortune. Having a heart attack is seen as a second chance disease, like no other. No one says, "My, you're lucky to have cancer of the lung," or "You're lucky to have diabetes," or "You're lucky to have MS," or "You're lucky to be showing signs of early-onset Alzheimer's."

Over the years I had read some of the cultural criticism of medicine, early Norman Mailer, middle Susan Sontag, their writings on cancer. They were precursors, though there always had been writers who had taken on disease: as a teenager, one of my favorite books had been Thomas De Quincey's *Confessions of an English Opium-Eater*. These days, you are what you have, both materially and medically.

Cancer seemed to fit the second half of the twentieth century. It was everywhere, even in Washington, D.C., when John Dean famously testified during the Watergate hearings of the early seventies, "There was a cancer—within—close to the Presidency."

Cancer multiplied cells and multiplied metaphors. But heart attacks became attached to the idea of rebirth, born again, renewal, more of a rite of passage, than a spiraling road to nowhere. One friend had written me that my heart attack was the Vietnam experience I had avoided. Well, I saw what he meant, but I knew it wasn't Vietnam.

Cancer seemed to be, what with the many treatments proliferating in the last decades, a catastrophic disease that quickly turned into a chronic one, as my older sister's then-husband, a physician, had put it. Death was often held at abeyance, at least for years beyond hope or expectation.

But given the transformations involved, the life of a cancer patient was a continual battle, skirmishes won or lost, periods of rest, and then, sooner or later, surrender.

Part of the "luck" of having a heart attack, of course, though it is often not directly expressed, is not dropping dead at the time of the attack. My Uncle Joe had narrated his death over the phone to his stepdaughter.

He had called her. She had called the ambulance. He lived in a rural district, and it took twenty minutes to get there. She called back, and he stayed on the phone until he fell dead. He told her he could hear the ambulance's siren, and then he said: "Oh, here it comes. . . ."

Nine years after my heart attack, two women professors died in classrooms here in South Bend within a few months of each other. Dropped in their tracks. In both cases, it wasn't the same sort of heart attack I had, but a slightly more complicated flaw and rupture. One was only forty-four, but she didn't know it was coming, a defect long undetected, though she had been to a doctor for tests, since she had been feeling poorly.

So why "lucky" springs from almost everyone's lips is because almost everyone knows someone who just dropped dead from a heart attack. If you didn't, you are one of the lucky ones.

Believe me, I felt lucky too. My life the fourteen months before my heart attack had not been riddled with happiness. Having a son was truly a joyful thing, profound and elating, but, in my case, it was mixed with anxiety and the turn of the century's chief cliché: stress. Oh, so much stress.

I called myself the founding member of OAF: the organization for Older American Fathers. My wife seemed to be in the right age range to have a child (early thirties), but I thought myself to be somewhat at the far reaches of the cycle. Not that I hadn't been exposed to older fathers, but they tended to be retreads, gents with new, very young wives, with grown children from earlier marriages, who couldn't stop procreating.

The previous summer we spent a little time with one such fellow, at a friend's summer place in New York state, on our way to Vermont, where I was to teach for a couple of weeks at the Bennington College summer writing workshops. Some twenty years earlier, I had read a novel about my friend's other guest, written by the guest's long-gone first wife—a depiction not at all complimentary. He did seem like an old roué to me, tall and lean: a cigarette holder personality, which kept him thin as a cigarette. His current wife was about four decades his junior, and he was looking to secure some work from my friend, a television producer. He had a new baby boy, as did we, but ours was a few months older. His was still a babe in arms, but not his arms. I don't think he glanced in the child's direction for the two days we were there, but his wife certainly doted on the tyke. It was noblesse oblige as fatherhood. He had done his part, supplied the sperm and, doubtless, the financial wherewithal.

But I was far from that epoch of detachment. Keeping Joe alive seemed to require constant vigilance. Joe's first months were marked by two things that marked me. The first was when my wife dropped him.

We were getting ready to travel to Kansas City for Thanksgiving, and I was in the house shutting off lights, when Teresa ran back in the house screaming, "I dropped him, I dropped him!" I didn't register the import of what she was saying, and I said, stupidly, "Dropped him. How could you drop him?" It was a question, not a rebuke, since I couldn't see just how one could drop a child.

"ON THE STAIRS! ON THE STAIRS!" she yelled.

The front door was still open, so I walked out the door, to pick him up, I suppose, though she had him in her arms. On the lawn a half-dozen bright orange persimmons, fruit her mother had sent her a few days before from California, were scattered about. I had noticed them earlier in a basket by the door. I turned back and took Joe from her. He was wearing a little knit cap, with a rolled edge, which had been some cushion, but there was dirt and cement dust on his forehead, which I began to brush away. He seemed stunned, but not unconscious. She had dropped him on the cement steps leading down from the front porch. I pictured Teresa trying to do too much at once, as was her wont, and somehow losing control of the basket of fruit and, in trying to catch it, letting go of Joe. She had been taking the fruit as a gift to a neighbor's house, it appeared.

She was on the phone with Joe's doctor—or, nurse, actually—and we set out to her office. Teresa was hysterical. I was still muttering, How could you have dropped him? though I already knew the answer.

In the car, Joe wasn't in his baby seat, but clutched in Teresa's arms, and there wouldn't be a way to correct that. Teresa found some comfort by yelling at me. Our marriage was not without stress. We got to the doctor's office, and Teresa, still sobbing, rushed in with Joe, while I trailed behind. We were sent immediately to a consultation room—a first—and the looks of the waiting patients were a mix of alarm and concern. Joe's cap was now off, and I explained how he had been wearing it before. There was a red mark with the fine lines of the concrete's rough finish still visible. Joe wasn't crying; he just appeared listless.

His doctor looked him over, gave him some liquid Tylenol, said the only thing to do was to observe him through the night and make sure he didn't worsen. She couldn't be certain if he had a concussion, and only time would tell.

Obviously, we couldn't fly to Kansas City that day, or perhaps not even the next. I didn't think there was much chance of getting different reservations, in any case.

We took him home, and, doubtless because of the Tylenol, he fell asleep. Every little while we looked at him, and he seemed to be sleeping peacefully enough. And certainly it was the longest stretch of hours he had ever slept. It was, I thought, the worst night of my life. When I awoke again from a couple hours of light sleep to check on him before dawn, I pulled myself out of bed as if out of some grave of my own making. What had we done to him?

I went into his room, and there he was, awake and needing to be changed. And he was smiling, gurgling, looking like his old self again. My heart soared. He was back! Seemingly without any lasting damage. Teresa was still asleep, so I changed him and that commotion must have awakened her, since she came into the bathroom. "See," I said, "it's Joe. He's OK."

We were both mightily relieved. And I was able to make new plane reservations, though we needed to leave from Chicago, not South Bend. I held him all the way on the bus to Midway airport and the plane ride to K. C. I was worried I was holding him too tightly, but the taste of his undoing had sunk so deeply into me that I felt I was reclaiming him, bringing him back from a great distance, by my protective embrace.

But I did not forget how I felt the morning I awoke after a fitful hour or so of sleep. Teresa seemed happy again. For a couple of weeks afterwards she and the other mothers around exchanged accounts of dropping their babies. It seemed to happen a lot—every mother had a story to tell.

–∿– The other thing, perhaps more important, happened right after his birth. He wasn't gaining weight. Teresa was breast-feeding him—all those La Leche-supporting-Lamaze classes—and losing weight herself simultaneously. We had been visited by a nurse a couple of days after we got home, so both Teresa and Joe could be checked, and they both seemed fine. Teresa had said to the nurse, pointing to me, "Check his blood pressure," and she did. As usual, it was high, 135/93.

The nurse looked concerned, and I said I knew about it and was seeing a doctor (let's let diet changes see if that can lower it, etc.). Joe was a big baby at birth, but it didn't take too long for him to grow thin, not fat. He needed food, and breast milk did appear to be insufficient, but before Joe actually got some formula, he was tested to see if he lacked some critical enzyme for absorbing fat. I remember the look in his eyes as I held him down to have some blood taken. But Joe didn't lack the enzyme. His failure to thrive, the diagnosis, was blamed on my wife's breast milk. We needed to go to one more

THE LUCKY DISEASE   63

doctor, who wasn't a huge fan of La Leche (she referred to La Leche's "cult of the boob" and "tyranny of the tit"), and she said, Give the boy some formula.

Why this hadn't been prescribed earlier, I don't know. I had, to my regret, gone along with the women who were professionally looking after Joe's welfare, along with my wife. It was a woman doctor, though, who finally said, Feed him. So I was able to feed him for the first time, and he gobbled up a bottle of formula in about three seconds (a hungry kid), and from then on he gained weight, still breast-feeding, but also having as much formula as he wanted. My wife's doctor, Joe's doctor, not the specialist we saw for another opinion, joked, "Oh, so he had an IQ of 160; now he'll only have 140. Who'll ever notice?"

I hadn't laughed. A month or so later Joe was dropped.

It had been a hard fourteen months prior to my heart attack, and keeping Joe alive didn't seem as easy as I would have thought, previous to his birth.

But keeping my own self alive, I hadn't realized, was a bigger problem.

—⋏— My career was still stalled, but I returned to Bennington and its summer writing workshops for a second stint the following summer. I was still in a state of ill-prepared fatherhood. I was pretty certain *Notts* would be difficult to sell (though not in England, I had thought, where it was set). I had been back in the Midwest for close to nine years since leaving the East Coast, and it was out of sight, out of mind, for the literary world of New York City. So I was happy to do the Bennington gig, since at least it was in the East Coast orbit. But I wasn't full of hope.

All my books were out of print, and I was out of shape. The first summer at Bennington, while I was embroiled in the NEA controversies of the time (1990), I was interviewed on New York City's progressive radio station, WBAI.

Joseph Papp, as I noted earlier, had become the leading figure in the New York–centric world of the NEA protest, and after my radio appearance even his stand altered and began to approach mine. Papp was on NPR saying that perhaps individual artists should take the money but that institutions should make "symbolic" protest by refusing it. I had pushed on WBAI and elsewhere the labor/management aspects of the protest, with all the producers like Papp, and the arts administrators and gallery owners and the like laying down the line, telling the individual artists what they should do. They all appeared to be more afraid of any legal repercussions than did the solo workers in the arts, the writers, painters, dancers, performers.

In any case, the entire episode had been thoroughly depressing. By my second summer visit to Bennington, the NEA had been largely gutted, its yearly budget reduced, and the arts community, so-called, was shown up as yet another cage overfilled with white mice who had resorted to cannibalism because of the desperate crowding. In America, where so few artists get any significant recognition, it is often just bloody tooth 'n' claw survival of the fittest on display, and the situation often seems to breed more personal animosity than you would find in other professions, even the law.

At Bennington there were some housing problems at first, and we had been assigned to a group living arrangement, but, with an eleven-month-old in tow, that seemed intolerable to me. I was able, after making a fuss, to get us other lodging, a small part of what purported to be one of Robert Frost's residences, the bulk of which remained empty and seemed quite charming. The nub end that we occupied had been turned into what was rudimentary dorm space, but it was ours alone.

Looking back at the year before one has a heart attack may be instructive, but it is usually not cheering. More than two vectors of my life were intersecting at an unhappy place. When it came to other writers whom I knew or associated with, a pattern had certainly developed.

I tended to identify with the underappreciated, not a difficult thing to do, since it is certainly made up of the largest numbers of authors. But it had started early in my writing life, with Edward Dahlberg, a man of much genius and much bile. Even earlier there had been Winfield Townley Scott, a poet who lived an entirely different sort of life (of ease in Santa Fe, New Mexico) from Dahlberg (living in genteel poverty in New York City), but Scott also de-spaired of his lack of attention and finally killed himself in the late sixties. I found myself in the orbit of any number of writers who had some fame, but no fortune, and then the fame flamed out. No per-manent orbit was achieved. Such a writer today is rarely elevated to the horizon of popular notice. It was a fifties and sixties kind of fame, not the sort that made an impression by the eighties and nineties.

There's much to be said both for and against this, and I myself have said and published quite a bit on it, which ended up in *Signs of the Literary Times*. But somewhere in the back of my own mind, I ac-knowledged that if you didn't have readers, if you couldn't locate an audience, it might not always be someone else's problem. Every once in a while I would be struck by doubt and remind myself that if the culture isn't listening, it is because you aren't telling it anything it wants to hear.

So as I cultivated my bitter garden, Teresa grew more and more alarmed with me. The first months of Joe's life (and the last months of her pregnancy) had taken, for other reasons, their toll on us. She was eleven years younger, and her career was beginning to take off as mine was becoming becalmed. Her book, which she had finished the year before at Bennington, had just been accepted by MIT Press, and she was about to receive tenure because of it. Things were start-ing to happen for her. I recognized the signs, better than I had in my own case.

I had no trouble walking (no angina) and didn't recognize any-thing as wrong, except the ferocious lack of sound sleep, although I knew I had to do something about my weight.

After Bennington we had planned to take a quick trip through my past to show off Joe. Teresa's past was on the West Coast; mine was on the East. So we went to Massachusetts, to South Hadley, to Cape Cod, Newport, Rhode Island, and New York City, before heading back to Indiana.

It was a melancholy trip, and it was hard at the time to account for why it caused me such anxiety. Driving, I suppose, was part of it, seeing so many people so quickly, and not seeing everyone I should have, given the limited time, and being presented with both the successes and failures of one's own past that display themselves on such a trip.

Joe had his first birthday party on St. Luke's Place at Jean Boudin's home. Leonard had died a couple of years previously, and my relationship with the Boudins since 1972 had been fraught with all sorts of conflicting emotions, since they, in many ways, had taken me on as a surrogate child, though they had two of their own, one now on the federal bench, another in a federal prison for her role in the Brink's robbery and murders, the Bedford Hills Correction Center.[1]

Only when we finally drove home did I seem to relax; at least, so I thought, my heart attack two short months away.

CHAPTER SEVEN
In My Own House

The first morning I woke up in my own house after the heart attack, home from the hospital, I hobbled downstairs to find the kitchen crowded. Not only were my parents and Teresa and Joe there, but a guy who had just installed glass block windows in the basement. I had contracted with him to do the job a month or so ago, and I had forgotten about it. He had taken measurements back then. It hadn't taken him long this Saturday morning to install the two windows. He seemed depressingly fit to me, a big, hearty, robust guy, with red suspenders, looking like an advertisement for the yuppie middle-aged craftsman. He lived on a street of gentrified city houses near us, a desirable street, quainter than ours.

I found the checkbook and wrote him a check. My parents were also leaving that day. They had been here ten days, almost my entire hospital stay, and wanted to get back to Kansas City, where my seven other siblings and a high number of grandchildren lived. When Teresa had called them, they had left a Florida vacation early to fly directly here, so they hadn't been home for nearly a month.

Teresa discovered that lightbulbs had started to burn out when she was gone, and she couldn't remember that happening before, or that toilet paper had run out, or that garbage began to pile up, and all that was new, too. My father replaced the burnt-out light bulbs and found the toilet paper and took out the garbage. Teresa had taken note of what she hadn't taken note of before.

So by late afternoon, the house was quiet again. Just Teresa, Joe, and me. I looked at pictures of Joe in his Halloween costume—he had been a bumblebee, with a padded belly. He still had long blond hair, not yet having his first real haircut. This Halloween his dad had been the scary heart patient. Teresa told me that when she had taken him to the hospital, people there thought I was going to die soon, since only in that circumstance were children that young allowed to visit the CCU. She also said that when my father had first taken Joe for a walk, he had started to cry when my father had put on a jacket of mine. He had cried so much that my father took it off and went outside for a walk in the cold with Joe without any coat.

My older sister Marita had sent from Kansas City a recently published book, *Doctor Dean Ornish's Program for Reversing Heart Disease,* which she inscribed, "May this book insure many more birthdays." Teresa had decided it would be twigs and berries from now on, something she had been pushing for years anyway. Since she grew up in Northern California and went to school at U.C. Berkeley, she had brushes before with vegetarianism and health food cuisine, so now it was to begin in earnest. Low fat, no fat, seemed to be the ticket. I was happy to eat anything. One of the appointments I was to keep soon would be the cardiology group's nutritionist, and that would be part of the rehab schedule I was to start. BlueCross BlueShield paid for about a dozen or so visits. The cardiologists had an exercise facility in their office building.

So life was to change, or, certainly, diet was to change.

That night, Teresa and I made love, not too athletically, though, I thought, tenderly. I suppose there was a good deal of sadness hovering about, accompanying the tenderness, or supplementing it. It had been Teresa's worst fear, or, if not the worst—that would have been a stroke, with me rendered an invalid—it was what she had feared, that I would become damaged goods (or more damaged goods).

She and I had many differences before the heart attack: she was always high energy, I not so high. I thought of myself, often described myself, as having stamina, but no energy. I envied those who were always said to possess "nervous" energy, because I seemed to have no nervous kind at all. If anything, I had nervous fatigue. But I was always steady, could go long hours. I had done so much manual labor when I was younger I always knew I was strong, and there came a time I thought the expense of energy in such things as jogging was some sort of luxury indulged in by those who had never had to work for a living, work with their backs, that is. But now I knew there was going to be a difference, and since things hadn't been so good the year before the heart attack, I didn't know how long it was going to take to bring me back to whatever the new "normal" would be.

I guessed six months, since guessing "six months" for anything always seemed safe.

I had lost ten pounds while in the hospital, so that was a start. Rehab would force some habit of exercise upon me, I presumed. Twigs and berries would certainly have their effect.

But I was certain our lovemaking had spent more energy than walking up stairs, even though our house had three stories; since I was back, I had already walked up and down the stairs a number of times.

There is a lot of alliteration, many *s*'s, when one is a heart patient: I found myself being sad, sorry, and scared. It's an odd triptych, but I suppose being scared is the largest panel, the one in the middle.

It was early November. Luckily, I was still on leave. An academic position is about the most flexible job one can have these days and was what allowed us to live up to our 50/50 childcare notions.

But the 50/50 was to be supplemented with some semiprofessional child care. Since my family lived in another state and Teresa's family lived on the West Coast, an extended family hadn't been available, except for the emergency care my parents had just provided. In Kansas City, my seven other siblings were able to avail themselves of grandparent services for their many offspring, my nieces and nephews. We arranged an interesting "nanny" (our independent contractor) for Joe. I think he had the only nanny who was in a higher income bracket than his mother and father. She was the wife of Teresa's department chair, and her kids were grown up and gone, and she wanted the work. That had been the arrangement that was about to begin, so it began a bit earlier than planned.

I had never been terribly body conscious. I was conscious that I was short. But, even at my heaviest, I didn't think much about being overweight. It didn't seem that foreign. I had still been strong, had no trouble walking or doing things. I had turned the attic into a study, filling the rafters with insulation, installing a skylight, using quarter-inch wafer board for walls. It had been a lot of work (and I certainly lost weight doing it) when we had moved into the current house, some two years earlier. And right after Joe was born, during my parents' first post-grandchild visit, I finished building a stockade fence around our backyard.

I had been on diets irregularly since I had been back in the Midwest. The most effective had been the Jean Harris Memorial Diet (my name for the Dr. Tarnower two-week high protein, low carbohydrate diet). The first time I had been on that, I had lost twenty pounds in two weeks; the second and third times, not so much, fifteen pounds, or so. But I would gain it back if the weight loss wasn't followed by a period of intense and sustained physical activity.

The first year of Joe's life certainly was exhausting, but it wasn't intense physical activity of the exercise sort, though it certainly was intense activity. Worry, no sleep, etc. But I wasn't body conscious. I just carried on. Teresa often suggested I lose weight. And, of course, there were those clippings from the *New York Times* of young men dying from heart attacks.

I've never been one for self-help literature—I had, actually, avoided it. Magazine pieces, though, I would occasionally read, and any heart-related information that would pass my way I would certainly glance at. If there was something on the radio, I would listen to it. Previous to the heart attack, I thought I had heard all the indicators there were for heart attacks. With each new one I would check it off as one I had. I think the last one I heard was "a lot of ear hair." Oh, yeah, I have that, too, I recalled saying to myself in front of the mirror as I was clipping off an excess of pesky ear hairs.

I didn't smoke, though, and I thought that significant. My mother did, and I happily didn't take it up, since I wasn't enamored of how it looked on her, as well as the overflowing cigarette ashtrays around our house in the 1950s. But the main reason was that I had decided that short people looked ridiculous smoking.

I don't know if that was being body conscious. More image conscious, I think. I never had angina, still couldn't tell you what that feels like now. But, upon returning home from the hospital, my body was certainly the most sensitive reed around. Any twinge or tremor felt direly significant. I was listening to my body far, far too attentively.

In a day or so I realized just being in bed for ten days or more had made me weak. I started walking as much as I could. Not too much, but around the neighborhood. I was out walking with Joe, and a car pulled up and stopped; a woman got out and ran up to me and hugged me, and, on her way to do that, I saw she was a former student of mine, one of the few older women who end up in a Notre Dame classroom, because courses were available to her as a member of the public relations staff. It wasn't exactly as if she had seen a ghost (one doesn't usually run up to embrace a ghost), but there was some sense of alarm to it. I remember Joe's expression, since he had never seen that happen before, a strange woman jump from a car to hug his dad. It was not a usual occurrence for me, either.

But it was clear that word had gone out around the school that I had had a heart attack. And since I hadn't been much on campus before it, my absence from it now might have seemed more total that I meant it to be. So I decided I should show up there soon, just so people wouldn't think I had died.

I had received cards, a few letters, some small gifts, all appreciated. The letters, especially, written by colleagues I actually hadn't spent that much time with. But I had to reply to them all, and I found myself doing some social reciprocating, as if having a heart attack was similar to getting married, or having a meaningful anniversary or promotion. In a way, it obviously was. But I also realized I hadn't gone through that many of these sorts of social rituals. Teresa and I had eloped.

I sent a memo to all my varied correspondents, and since it captures my tone of voice at the time, I reproduce it below. I also included a drawing of my heart, on which I circled the sites of blockages and buildup, identifying them with the names of my books (see Figure A).

TO: Those in the loop
FROM: W. O'Rourke
RE: Heart as text
DATE: 18 November 1991

By way of explanation, I wanted you to know I had a heart attack on October 26th, sitting in Notre Dame's football stadium before the USC game. As such things go, it wasn't bad. It appears I have healthy arteries for a sixty-five year old. In order to reach that age I have to change my ways. OK, OK, I promise. I actually think the cause of the attack was Clarence Thomas. I was, as the expression goes, heartsick over that display of the body politic. I'm better now, almost "normal", doing what I'm told. Since I'm on leave this semester, I can move slow. Teresa and Joe make things easier. I'm trying to unknot *Notts,* which I still hope to have finished by January. Sorry for this news, and how. Now, with the picture of my heart, you know more about me than I knew about me.

Being on leave was fortuitous, not so much for my own work, but for recovering from a heart attack. One singular consequence was that there were no adverse financial consequences. I am an exception to the rule.

When I was in the hospital, Teresa said that, upon returning from getting a cup of coffee, she had run into a young woman who had taken the bus—which had cost her $100—to see her father before his operation but had to leave since it took so many days to get here—and therefore get home—before the surgery took place. She told Teresa she would lose her job if she didn't get back.

My economist wife pointed out that the young woman's situation was typical. Everyone, it was clear, had more job costs than I had. I was on leave. In that way alone my experience seemed to be unique.

Heart as text:

CARDIAC CATHETERIZATION DIAGRAM

AORTA

RIGHT CORONARY ARTERY DOMINANT

Teresa + Joe

Naval

AORTA

LEFT VENTRICLE

% = % obstruction

40%

RIGHT CORONARY

OK

LEFT MAIN

Notts

CIRCUMFLEX

OBTUSE MARGINAL

Idle Hands

ANTERIOR DESCENDING

100%

The Harrisburg 7

The Meekness of Isaac

Criminal Tendencies

BlueCross BlueShield paid over $20,000 for my care but never sent me an itemized bill, just a letter claiming they had somehow "saved" me money.[1] And I didn't need to resume work immediately. It didn't take me too long, however, to feel guilty about Teresa getting up early and taking care of Joe in the morning, while I slept another hour or two, except for the two days she taught classes. After a few weeks, we began to resume more shared child care, but it took nearly six months to get back to where it had been, 50/50 or, rather, 75/75.

I had received some generational solidarity from our nanny (she was closer in age to me than to Teresa), who said I had been doing too much shopping and looking after Joe before the heart attack and that had been a contributing factor, which I don't think was the case (in the way she meant it), but I took comfort from any notice of what I had been doing. Just as I took comfort from the displays of shock or affection from people I knew.

But, after a few days, rehab was on the horizon, and that I looked forward to: supervised exercise. I liked the idea of being looked after. That seemed new.

⌐⌐ The cardiology group had its offices a couple of blocks from the hospital where I had been treated. For South Bend, it was a rather modern-looking building, something usually found in the woods of Colorado, a lot of vaulted glass and redwood stained lumber. It was, in its way, a cardiology mall. I would see my doctors there, and I would also use the rehab wing. In the large open waiting area there was a good-sized decorative water fountain, putting off watery negative ions and other good vibes. Free coffee and donuts(!). It was New Age decor, except for the donuts. I stuck to water, from a water fountain.

For rehab we were all wired up, harnessed with a belt carrying a portable transmitter, sending our heart rhythms to a nurse's station monitor. One of the nurses looked like an aerobics instructor; the others did not.

I did ten minutes on a treadmill at set speeds, ten minutes on a stationary bicycle, then free weights, pulleys, and one machine for arm and upper-body strength. I was the youngest person in the room, aside from the nurse who could have been an aerobics instructor.

I had seen all the machines before, except for the arm-strengthening device, which did look like something you would find in a doctor's office. But I could see immediately the usefulness of the rehab: all the machines looked faintly dangerous. I certainly needed to be desensitized. It was a pleasure to drive again, since I had driven here. But the treadmills somehow seemed ominous, as if they were all programmed to give stress tests, as if each bit of exercise were some sort of test. But we started slow, and the nurses kept watch.

I contemplated my fellow rehabbers. They all seemed to be close to sixty, or over that. Most overweight; it looked like Irish stew, white, creamy, potatoes, bleached out lamb, and for color, some carrot-orange hair. It definitely looked like an ethnic demographic. But it must also be Polish, or other Eastern European (again, both sides of my family), a slew of nightmare relatives all pumping their little bits of iron.

Though of course black people have heart attacks, they were not with this group, or they didn't have the same good insurance. There was one fellow who didn't fit the pattern; I had seen him at school, a math professor I thought, and he didn't look good, though he was definitely not overweight. He had what to me looked like Kaposi's sarcoma, but, if he was here, it must be something heart related. I never found out. (He died in 1998.) I didn't exchange anything but pleasantries with the fellow walkers and bikers. Everyone seemed fairly serious, and, given what I was learning about heart-attack profiles, I wasn't surprised that these folks, like me, weren't the most outgoing group. Introversion seems to run in heart patients, or, rather, the habit of keeping things in. Apart from the whirring machines, there was a lot of silence in the rehab room.

Having a child drives your empathy quotient way up, and having a heart attack does too. It forces some sort of patience on you, some sort of acceptance. So I would arrive, get hooked up, do my forty-five minutes of exercise, and depart.

The interview with the nutritionist was scheduled, and my wife came along for this conference (it was presumed she would be doing the cooking.) The nutritionist produced the diet recommended by the American Heart Association (AHA), and my wife was aghast, having done her own readings and research on the subject. The nutritionist's explanation for the high amount of fat and meat allowed on the AHA diet was that more restrictive diets wouldn't be tolerated by the patients. But Teresa had become a Dr. Dean Ornish convert (Ornish was the creator of a program he claimed could reverse heart disease), and she wanted the fat portion dropped as close to zero as possible.

I recalled the two meals I had had before the heart attack. The triggering devices, as I began to think of them. One was on Thursday, two nights before my MI. We had gone to a faculty dinner party given by a friend and colleague of Teresa. In fact, Teresa was responsible for her having her job—and her present boyfriend, also a colleague in the economics department. And for the house she was living in. She had bought the smaller one we had near the campus when we sold it. Candy was also a Berkeley grad, but she wasn't into twigs and berries, or even granola, but into what was really sweeping the landscape of yuppiedom at the time, even in the most progressive circles: gourmet cooking, no fear of fat, tasty and attractive, something out of the Alice Waters/Chez Panisse school of dining.

So there was a succulent, rare, blood-running lamb, oil-drenched sautéed vegetables, some unbelievable chocolate torte, and Teresa, trying to cut down her intake, kept giving me what she wouldn't eat, which I gladly did. I got quite a bit of pleasure from eating. A wonderful meal.

The next night, we went to a bar, Albert's, a regular Friday outing, where members of the English and theology departments got together for talk. Then we went to the Sandeens' house for dinner, spaghetti with meat sauce.

But Teresa was sure it had been Candy's lamb and chocolate torte dinner that was the killer. There's a medical description of what an infusion of just such a high-fat, high-everything meal produces: thromboxane, which, it is claimed, causes the arteries to constrict and blood to clot more quickly. When I took my brisk walk to Notre Dame Stadium the following Saturday, that's what had been sloshing around in my system.

〰 There was a small amount of competition, as well as coopera-
tion, between my two doctors, the cardiologist and the internist. But
it was more or less settled with my cardiologist's remark, "We'll let
him take care of your lipids." My cardiologist had put me on a cholesterol-lowering drug, Mevacor, as he left my room right before I had
been released. My new internist had taken me off of it.

I was put on a large dosage of Lopid: 600 milligrams twice a day.
That was to deal with my high triglycerides, which did not seem to
be affected by my new diet. My cholesterol, which had dropped because of the diet, remained very low, barely over a hundred, even
after I was off the Mevacor. My good cholesterol wasn't high, though.
Lopid was supposed to help raise that level, eventually. Is this a drug
for life?, I asked my internist. He said yes.

I was taking a low dose of Cardizem (60 milligrams), a calcium
channel blocker. My blood pressure was low (110/74), so I wasn't
taking any additional medication for that. I took a baby aspirin, 81
milligrams. So at the moment, my drugs were split between the doctors: Cardizem from the cardiologist, Lopid from my internist, and
aspirin from over the counter.

None of the drugs felt in any way recreational. During my initial
visit with the internist, I mentioned my "no energy, but stamina"
equation and that I didn't know how I should be feeling at forty-six,
since I had never been forty-six before (my birthday had just come
and gone). I did feel out of sorts, or certainly altered. He offered,
turning away at the same time, that having a heart attack is something "life changing," and if I thought it necessary, he advised, some
people see a psychologist afterwards.

My attitude toward shrinks had always been standoffish. I knew
a few socially over the years, and given my life as a writer, I thought
I had been living an almost too examined life, especially since a lot
of my fiction was directly autobiographical. But his mention of that
recourse was perfunctory. And so was my response to it.

I continued to lose weight, and the exercise at rehab picked up. I
still listened for every twinge or gurgling message. Having never detected any feelings of angina, I tended to be most alarmed at any
sensation that was near or around my chest.

My cardiologist, during a scheduled visit, announced that they had just gotten a new machine and I was to be one of its first benefi-ciaries. So I was hooked up to it, some sort of supersensitive EKG apparatus, though it was to detect something more specific and hard to pin down. It was clear from the nurses operating it that they were just learning how to use it. But after a few tries, they got some sort of reading. I was told to be very still, and I saw myself as a good pa-tient, so I complied.

I had noticed that a lot of the medical world had become what I termed "harem professions." Dentist offices were almost always that way (unless the dentist was a woman). You would find one man (the dentist) and about ten women working for him. The cardiology group was similar. Five male doctors and about thirty women doing their bidding. So the nurses would shave my chest, manipulate my body, fuss over me. It was the closest I had ever been to a massage parlor.

A few days later I was called to come back in and take another test. In the intervening days I don't know if their skills had pro-gressed much, or if they had other people to test the machine on, since I thought it was the machine that was being subjected to the test, more than the subject being tested. But after a while and a few tries, they thought they had gotten another satisfactory set of readings.

I was told to make an appointment with the cardiologist who was the electrician of the group, Dr. V. C., the one who had treated me at the emergency room. He had the various readouts in front of him and said, "Well, this shows some anomalies, some irregulari-ties." He proceeded to describe an apparatus, not a pacemaker, but something more elaborate that could be stuck under my skin, wired into my heart, and turned on if I ever fell into a heart rhythm that was life-threatening. But, finally, he wasn't sure these were the most convincing readings, and for now he thought it best just to see if it wouldn't work out by itself. The progress I thought I had been making seemed to be set back, and the small twinges I felt began to take on more ominous tones than I hitherto had ascribed to them.

I went off to my rehab the next day, none too chipper, and mentioned to the nurse what tests I had just been taking, and she said, "Oh, my guys [meaning us in rehab] get funny readings all the time." She pointed to her machine's monitor. Then she said she asked them how many cups of coffee they had before they came over today, and they'd tell her, three, four, and that's usually the reason. I recalled the nurse who told me about the pain I would feel if the tPA worked. Nurses will often supply information your doctor will neglect to tell you.

When I was called to come in once more for the same test I had had three times already, I didn't drink any coffee for twenty-four hours before the test. They got their reading a bit quicker this time.

A month or so later, after yet another test (that new machine was getting a workout, along with my BlueCross account), with no coffee for a day, I saw my plumber cardiologist. He looked over my records and said, Yes, I see that you were advised to wait and see, which turned out to be good advice, since you don't seem to have the problem we feared. He said it with disinterest and just a trace of disappointment, since he certainly was the action-oriented one, the doc who wanted to do something, with a penchant for and facility with hardware.

CHAPTER EIGHT

The Medically Compromised

There is as much literature for the spouse of the medically compromised as there is for the patient. The heart attack sufferer is no different. I almost typed "victim," instead of "sufferer," which puts the correct cultural spin on the conventional wisdom. What is the person a "victim" of? His or her lifestyle? Genetics? The diet and exercise predilections of the typical American in a sedentary suburban culture of fast food and no sidewalks?

"Sufferer" is a bit more neutral, in so far as we all suffer the consequences of our own acts, including the more evanescent nature of who we are. So Teresa's view of my heart attack was, in many ways, unlike my own. She was more a victim of it than I was. Though we certainly shared a degree of fright. But she was scared in a different way.

Three years before my heart attack a friend had published a book (under a pseudonym, Maggie Strong) called *Mainstay: For the Well Spouse of the Chronically Ill.* Her husband, my friend, too, had suffered from MS (Multiple Sclerosis). I had moved from the East Coast before its really debilitating effects had set in. Since some heart attacks are the "lucky" disease, I do not grow progressively worse; at least, not in someone's—my—system of estimation. I do grow older.

But my young wife found in my heart attack the emblem of all her very worst fears. It's hard for someone who embodies vitality to be the consort of one who has almost lost it. And her vitality is her hallmark. Her beauty is in her animation. It was one more thing thrown into the mix of a marriage that hadn't undergone much scrutiny—on my part.

Teresa wasn't rosy about a number of things, two being where we lived and what we did. Her position at the university was her first job. She wanted it not to be her last job. She had dreamed, more than I then knew, of living on the East Coast. I had lived on the East Coast. It was part of our age differences. What we saw as necessary for our lives was somewhat out of sync. But, when I got married, I realized that she would need a life she hadn't yet lived, in order to get on in the world. She would need to go places and do things.

So shortly after we were married, she got a Bunting Fellowship, and we went to Cambridge, Massachusetts, to live while I commuted back to Notre Dame. I knew she needed to do that sort of thing, to have the ability, the freedom, to seize whatever opportunities that came along. And I didn't find it difficult to accommodate to the situation. By being single all those years, I had had a lot of freedom.

After Joe was born, she certainly wasn't going to let a baby slow her down any more than necessary. She knew that more than one would slow her down. The day after we got back from the hospital with Joe—the day after he was born—she went to summer school graduation to hood a student of hers who was getting his Ph.D. After the heart attack, after the rehab set in, our old routines came back, though I was still cut a little slack. At least, I thought so.

But Teresa had a new opportunity: she took a leave from Notre Dame to work for the AFL-CIO in Washington, D.C. This time she would commute; I wouldn't be traveling there as much as I had done when she was in Massachusetts. Joe's life would make that impossible. Underneath the temporary employment while she was on leave was her hope that she would get the job permanently and we would somehow all move to Washington. I didn't think that likely, but I found a way to free up a semester down the road, by teaching a double load the semester before, in case the job was extended another six months. That seemed to be something I could agree to.

It also seemed to be some sort of public statement that I had re-covered from the heart attack. When I appeared back on campus, after my leave was over, the department cut my teaching load by one class—a medical dispensation—for a semester. I had managed to send a number of my colleagues to doctors for checkups. A col-league's husband's checkup had lead to immediate bypass surgery. He was gallant enough to thank me for "saving his life."

One "lucky" heart attack does have a beneficial ripple effect in the local medical community, regardless of whatever the underlying ailment is. A lot of people run to doctors. It's good for business all around.

But, after that semester passed, the freshness of my calamity grew stale, and soon things returned to old routines. Cancer is more difficult. Depending on what type of cancer it is, a lot of people go into a premature mourning, already writing off the person as going, going, gone. There is a slow withdrawal, as if the person is fading from a photograph. I had been part of that process before, I real-ized; I'd done it to people I know, or knew. It happens especially if you don't see the person on a regular basis. I had reached a certain age when almost everyone looks vaguely familiar, since you have seen or known so many people. I think it comes from having lived half a life, which I had, if I was lucky, at forty-six.

Mortality becomes a central issue following a heart attack, espe-cially for the first year afterward. One doesn't need a skull on a desk to inspire such reflection; any picture of a heart will do. Even pass-ing by a pile of frozen Cornish game hens in a supermarket will do. You dwell on the people you know who have died, died young, or even died old, since there is that odd line (when? seventy-five? eighty? sixty-five?) one crosses where it seems that one has lived a full allotment, a full life. Anything beyond becomes gravy (Ray-mond Carver's word), and when someone dies beyond that line, it doesn't seem so out of the ordinary.

The early deaths, though, are another matter. Suicides are mixed with volition. And leave both bereavement and wonderment be-hind. Why, why? Friends, the children of friends. Each case be-comes a monument to futility. And the medical deaths. A monument to what? Bad luck? When Teresa was having miscarriages and it seemed as if she might not carry a pregnancy to term, I would feel some empathy for the people who go to such extreme lengths to get pregnant—mainly because it was one of those things that seemed so simple, since there are people for whom it is no chore. It is the position of people with disabilities; difficulty encountered where most encounter none. I recall when curbs were first being ripped up a couple of decades ago to make inclines for wheelchairs. It seemed both a long time in coming and finally an acknowledgment that life could be made easier for everyone, not just the statistical majority.

So it appeared there could be the fertility challenged. But we didn't turn out to be that couple. And friends with cancer fell into a statistical minority. Throat cancer killed a friend of mine in her forties. She never smoked when I knew her, and I had known her for two decades. My friend Ernie Sandeen died of complications of throat cancer, both the disease itself and the methods of treatment, but he was in his eighties and had smoked a pipe all his adult life.

Ernie I saw a lot of, since he was in town. Sharli Land, my friend with throat cancer, I didn't see, since she lived in another state, though I once almost made a visit there, but didn't—something I often found myself doing or, rather, not doing. Jean Boudin died of cancer. She was in her eighties; Inez died of cervical cancer in her fifties. After a certain age, one finds oneself in a room populated with dead friends.

Then there are the suicides, another sort of the medically compromised: young women, one in her forties, the other still in her twenties. The son of a friend, a shotgun pressed against his head.

The living, of course, carry the dead forward, with us; this is why they are never gone entirely, except for those whom no one carries, and I suppose there are too many of them to count.

The acute preciousness of life one easily feels after a heart attack wanes. Though not completely. Teresa had begun to travel frequently. At first for a book on the pension fund of the operating engineers' union. Then for six months because of her job with the AFL-CIO in Washington. She would come home on the weekends. Most weekends. She was young and could do that, I thought. During spring break week, Joe and I went there, and we made a couple of weekend visits along the way too.

But it certainly rearranged the workload, let the heart attack recede into something like history, since Joe and I spent so much time with each other. I continued to desire calm and routine, which Teresa's commuting periodically allowed. She saw all that as another version of inaction, death. For her calm routine was the whiteness of the whale, something to be feared; for me, it seemed vital. The steady pumping heart. There are a lot of difficulties with this sort of commuting. One was that when Teresa came home, she wanted to party, to celebrate, for us to make a big fuss. We just wanted to fold her into the routine. Mom's home.

My way of coping was not hers. (Still isn't, for that matter.) But I saw all that time with Joe as compensatory, for the first couple of months afterwards, when I was recuperating.

Joe and I fell into the habit of watching "I Love Lucy" during the months Teresa commuted. (No Cartoon Network on our cable then, only Nickelodeon.) He was only four, but he laughed and laughed at the jokes and the slapstick humor. When I read to him, I sometimes was so tired that I would begin to nod off, and he would elbow me to wake up, wake up, so I could finish whatever Berenstain Bears book I was reading. It was a weird time, largely private, being a single father. Teresa's job was as public as my routine was private. She was with the movers and shakers, and I often required Joe to shake me to keep up and awake. Though he was reading by himself, he still wanted me to read to him. As it had happened with his so-called toilet training. At his nanny's house he used the toilet for a couple of weeks before he would use one at home.

I was plodding on with my career. After many attempts, I had found a publisher to take a collection of previously published short nonfiction pieces called *Signs of the Literary Times*. During the two years that took, Teresa kept informing me of the unlikelihood of finding a publisher. Finally, a university press accepted it, not to my complete surprise. I had finished *Notts*, the coal mining novel; no publisher for that had yet appeared. But I pushed on.

I was definitely not like Anthony Burgess, who, after some medical emergency, was told that he only had a few months to live, so he banged out a few novels during that time, including *Clockwork Orange*. Because of what has occurred in the literary world, the writers who became famous in the 1960s are still famous, and, because of advances in medicine, they are for the most part still alive, though of the triptych of Saul Bellow, Norman Mailer, and Joseph Heller, only Mailer is still with us.

But that World War II generation does seem to have been long-lived, doubtless because of all the significant history they have lived through. So many changes, so many different lives. But a literary life is not always the most life-affirming, if one has not achieved sufficient fame to have readers, a sense of being what one wants to be: a writer who is read.

The Reagan-Bush, Bush-Quayle era had come to an end in late '92, while I was recuperating from the heart attack, and the election of the baby-boomer, draft-dodger president lifted my general spirits—always good for a heart patient. I had never thought an anti–Vietnam War protestor would' be elected president. Hey, I thought, anything's possible now.

Clinton had good luck. The viperish Ross Perot seemed to hate George Bush without end, and Perot's presence in the '92 race helped Clinton slip on by into the presidency. And George Bush had made a fatal error when he selected Dan Quayle to be his veep. Bush had begun to show his age by the end of his first term (puking on the Japanese premier, his heart arrhythmia, other reported problems), and that made the possibility of President Quayle more likely, a troubling thought to a lot of Americans.

Teresa was commuting to Washington for the AFL-CIO during the midterm elections of 1994 and watched with amazement as twelve thousand people lost their jobs when the Republicans won the Congress for the first time in forty years. Democratic consultants were being kicked off the rising ship of Gingrichites. The streets were filled with these well-dressed castaways. It was quite a shakeout.

While Teresa was gone during the week, Joe and I did the cooking, which involved using the microwave quite a bit. Since I was the leading edge of my population cohort (the baby boom begins officially in 1946; I was born in December 1945), I was aided in my reduced fat diet by Madison Avenue and the great processed food companies. The strict twigs and berries of the first three years post-

MI had lessened, and I ate a lot of Healthy Choice frozen low-fat dinners. So my weight stayed pretty constant, since the portions were small and I didn't drink at all when Teresa was gone. Joe, alas, hadn't turned into an omnivore. He announced when he was about four that he was a vegetarian, and he didn't get that vocabulary from me. But if you are what you eat, Joe was a grilled cheese sandwich. His diet had been more varied when I used to feed him from glass jars, but there are worse eccentricities he could have displayed.

Teresa's stint with the AFL-CIO came to an end without my, or our, having to decide to move or not to move to Washington. It turned out she was overqualified for the position. She needed a staff, rather than to be on staff.

So by the summer of '95, we were a nuclear family once again, though Teresa still traveled quite a bit. She had become an international expert in her field, and she was in demand around the world. Then President Clinton appointed her to a federal agency, and we went under FBI scrutiny for six months. That was, for me, an unlikely turn of events, inviting the FBI into our life, giving them permission to look anywhere they wished. Supposedly, they didn't investigate me, and I took that assurance at the Feds' word, since what I knew—and had written about the Hoover-era agency—would not make simple incompetence look out of place. Anyway, Teresa had no problems.

My yearly physical exam consisted mainly of a stress test, and I kept passing that. The only medical change in my condition had occurred about a year after the MI, when my blood pressure began to rise. The dosage of Cardizem was raised, and when that didn't immediately lower it, I was put on a blood pressure pill, Zestril, which dropped it like a stone.

The medicines I had been taking then held constant for a number of years: Lopid, Cardizem, Zestril, and a baby aspirin every day (the Lopid twice a day).[1]

South Bend, home of Notre Dame, had long been culturally deprived, in so far as it lacked any substantial bookstores. So when Barnes & Noble finally built a store here, it was a cultural boon, not a community calamity. And it also provided students a place to go till eleven at night where they didn't have to drink. When I had left the Midwest for the East Coast in 1968, I was convinced the Midwest was at least ten years behind the rest of the country in certain ways. By the nineties, it was perhaps only five years behind. The first real coffee house, the beatnik sort, opened only a few months before the Barnes & Noble superstore.

Since these new bookstores are actually museums of sorts, where patrons go to "look" at the books, I was able to start looking through various medical guides and took some interest in the descriptions of my medications. My internist, in a moment of real candor, once described all my medications as poisons, but ones with beneficial results.

But before I read all the fine print, I had another experience that took me to the emergency room. This time, in 1995, I took myself.

My medicine routine had been to take my blood pressure–lowering pill, the Zestril, at night, right before bed, along with the second of my twice-a-day Lopid (600 milligrams). When I was given the Zestril (10 milligrams), no one had suggested a time to take it; I was told just to take it once a day.

So I took it, along with a large dose of Cardizem (300 milligrams, another one-a-day drug) around eleven at night, or shortly before bedtime. One night I awoke around one or two to go to the bathroom. I can't recall if I had drunk a lot of liquid, more than usual, that night, since I would usually wake up at five for the same purpose. I probably had. So I got up quickly and walked none too steadily into the unlit bathroom. And right before I started to urinate, my legs gave out from under me. I didn't pass out. I know that, since I was conscious of what happened. I started to fall, knocking into the toilet, which caused the toilet seat (which was up) to fall forward. I dropped face first onto it as it was falling shut. I bounced off it and hit the floor. I got myself up (the use of my legs had returned) and urinated as I had planned to and walked back into the bedroom. I hadn't turned any lights on, so it was fairly dark, except for some light coming up the stairwell from the front hall, where a light burned on through the night.

Teresa, having been awakened by the noise, asked me what happened. I told her. She laughed nervously. Then I felt my face, or something made me lift my hand to my face, and it felt wet. So I got up again and went back into the bathroom, this time turning on a light.

My upper lip and chin were covered in blood. I looked closer and saw a deep cut, a slash above my upper lip over an inch long and more than a quarter of an inch deep. Given its size, I was surprised that there wasn't more blood.

I returned to the bedroom after cleaning my face a bit and told Teresa I needed to go to the hospital, since it looked like a bad cut, not one of the Band-Aid variety. She got up and confirmed my diagnosis.

Since Joe was asleep and I didn't feel impaired, I decided to drive to the emergency room. I had been back to it with Joe a couple of times since my heart attack, once for an episode of croup in the middle of the night when Teresa had been out of town and once during the afternoon when Joe cut his chin and Teresa had been teaching.

Joe cut his chin—or, actually, right under his chin—three times in all. The first time was in South Dakota, where Teresa had been lecturing. We had breakfast with the organizers of the event, and one was an emergency room doctor. I had gone up to our room to get our coats (we were on our way to see the presidents carved in stone on Mount Rushmore), and when I returned, I found Teresa and a woman examining Joe's chin, from which dangled a strand, a tiny blob, of his own yellow fat. He had been standing on a chair and had tumbled off. We got to the emergency room, and it was the same doctor who came out to treat Joe with whom we just had breakfast. The second time Joe had been spinning around in the hallway, when his nanny had brought him home, and he had pulled his coat down over his shoulders and tripped. With his arms locked to his side by his coat he fell onto the hardwood floor like a toppled tree. His chin was split again.

All this chin splitting had taken a toll on me, trying to comfort him while he received stitches. (The third was the least serious.) So this time I was happy he could sleep and Teresa could too. I went to the same hospital emergency room I had been taken to in the ambulance.

I was cleaned up again, and a doctor, a young man, stitched me up. I told him what happened, and they ran an EKG on me, but he said it could have been any number of things. One theory had to do with some effect of the start of urination, which can trigger, so he said, some muscle failure. But I hadn't started to urinate. I didn't question his diagnosis; I just wanted to be back home.

When I got home, I saw what looked like a real Frankenstein kind of stitching. The cut was a very straight line above my lip on my left side, and he joined it together with four long stitches, spaced like guitar strings, each about an inch long themselves. I had been expecting a sewn seam.

Later in the morning I discovered why he had done it that way. I awoke with the stitches feeling very taut, as if they might snap. My upper lip was very swollen. I supposed they had to be long to have some give. I called the hospital, and the nurse said that the swelling was expected. But they hadn't told me to expect it. Getting the right information is often hit or miss. When so much is available, so much slips by.

I was teaching that day, and, though the students looked at me strangely, no one asked. I supplied that it had been a hard night, rather than saying I collided with a toilet seat, wanting to keep some air of mystery about their creative writing professor.

I went to my internist to have my stitches taken out, as I had been instructed. It seemed to have healed fairly well. The scar was a very fine line.

So I went through the description of the event again, and my internist supplied the same explanation as the emergency room doctor. Back to that magical moment of urination that can cause the loss of stability in the legs.

It happened again a couple of years later. The same thing. But this time I fell sideways, not straight down, and, once again, didn't lose consciousness.

Bam, bam, bam, I hit the side of our old cast iron bathtub, the sort with claw feet. I bounced from the tub to the toilet, smacked hard. This time Teresa came into the bathroom as I was attempting to stand up. When she was behind me, she grabbed me, thinking I was falling again, but I was just trying to get my balance from the battering I had just taken between tub and toilet, not from whatever made me fall in the first place.

I wasn't bleeding anywhere, so I just got back into bed, feeling, as before, humiliated and puzzled, as well as hurt. In the morning my face was black and blue, one side especially. Again, my students just stared, but they were a different class, different students.

It did look as though I had been beaten up, but I had done the beating.

This time I didn't see any doctors, although I was going to mention it to my doctor when I saw him for my annual checkup. When I did, he didn't seem too concerned about it. I looked "normal" again, by that time.

After that, not so long ago, I finally read all the small print on the Zestril information sheet, and one of the warnings contained a description of just what had occurred to me. It advised: You may get dizzy if you rise quickly from a sitting or lying position.

Well, it would have been helpful for someone to have mentioned the medication I was taking as a possible cause. I also had discovered that with these one-a-day pills, the largest part of the dosage is released fairly soon after it is taken. So I moved my time of ingestion from right before bed till around noon, figuring I was most awake then and wouldn't likely start to pass out, since I wouldn't have the sudden disruption of posture, from lying down to standing up quickly, that seems to trigger the event. I also implemented a low-tech way to solve the problem. If I awoke during the night, I sat down to urinate, instead of standing.

But, my question was—and still is: if in this small way the blind still lead the blind (I am both blind sides at once), what other things born out of ignorance am I doing to myself, unaided by professionals who miss remarking about the possible outcomes of what I have been told to do, told to take?

CHAPTER NINE

The Subject Turned to Health

In the spring of 1992 I was speaking with the writer Harold Brodkey, and, after we touched on some literary matters, the subject turned to health, since, by then, I had been doing nearly a half-year's worth of my sort of private cardiac rehab. He expressed some surprise at my tale of having a heart attack at forty-five. We talked about diets. Brodkey suggested the name of a macrobiotic master in Manhattan I should contact. I had been on the twigs and berries diet, almost no fat, but heavy on carbs and sugar.

Brodkey seemed very relaxed, almost serene. He had given a reading at the university earlier in the evening. We had talked about his long-, *long*-awaited novel, *The Runaway Soul,* which had finally been published the previous year. I asked if he thought he had waited too long, missing, by about a decade, the literary world's appetite for his rich, lyrical sensibility. No, he said, he thought not. He seemed to have no regrets, only literary certainties, especially about his own writing's merit.

We had some mutual acquaintances from the time I lived in Manhattan. When Brodkey's most famous short story "Innocence" was first published in the *New American Review* (number 16) in 1973, I remembered bantering about it with my girlfriend at the time, another young writer like me. Brodkey had described an elaborate act of lovemaking, which, eventually, led the woman involved to orgasm. I thought it was, though highly detailed, somewhat strained, and I was making light of it, thinking I was talking to an adept, a woman who didn't require such a 12-step program to completion. She made a remark that was laced with doubt and irritation, and, for the first time, I realized all was not as I had thought.

Back then, in the early seventies, it was still an older generation's literary world. I had another friend who worked at the *New Yorker* and who had divorced one of its prominent short-story writers, and she had gatherings of folk who were Brodkey's generation and older, guys like Milton Klonsky, who were known to the writers of New York, but not known anywhere else. At the time, Brodkey was one of those writers. He had published a slim volume of stories much revered by his compatriots. "Innocence," however, because of its sexual depiction, eventually brought him to the attention of a younger generation. But, because of my friend, he had already come to my attention.

So I was happy to talk with him some twenty years later, though, given his doting on macrobiotics, I wondered what ailed him. He didn't seem frail, but had the porcelain-like skin tones that often make cancer patients look so fragile. He was not forthcoming about any of that, but the question did pass through my mind, What does he have?

A few months later he announced in the *New Yorker* that he had AIDS.

Other memories came back when I read about that, things I had forgotten the evening in '92 when I had spoken with him. That a friend and I had gone to the Manhattan Theater Club a year or two after "Innocence" appeared, to hear Brodkey give a reading. I recalled sitting there, in that small theater, when a grumpy guy, somewhere in his sixties, got up to leave. He charged Brodkey with all manner of blasphemy, in the same vein Philip Roth's co-religionists had complained about his novel *Portnoy's Complaint,* damning it as filled with anti-Semitism.

What I remember was saying to my friend that Brodkey's story, performed by him, seemed like some sort of drag performance, an act of cross-dressing. That he wanted to be a woman and that's why he got into the meticulous descriptions so wholeheartedly. My friend looked at me dubiously.

In Brodkey's book about dying from AIDS, *This Wild Darkness,* he doesn't go on about macrobiotic diets—his doctor wants him to gain weight, however that's achieved.

Health has always been a literary subject, and dying even more so. Heart attacks don't turn up in fiction as much as one would think. Gail Godwin has recently published a Valentine Day's volume called *Hearts,* which covers some of the literary ground. Philip Roth's novel *Counterlife* makes use of a bypass operation in its plot but does not describe it at length.

I had read John Updike's *Rabbit at Rest* (it had come out in 1990) a year before my own heart attack. He describes one there, and, though when I read it at the time it seemed perfectly adequate, looking at it again makes one realize how little true experience one needs to have to make an untrue one accepted as real. Updike's novel is broken up into three sections, "FL," "PA," and "MI." The first was set in Florida, the second in Pennsylvania, and, when I first read the novel, I kept wondering why the last was called Michigan, since it didn't take place there. It was only after my heart attack did I realize MI stood for myocardial infarction, a heart attack.

Updike is well known for his proclivity for extensive research, especially in his Rabbit books. He needed to find out how a Toyota dealership was run, and doubtless he did research into the angiogram and angioplasty described in the novel. He has both procedures happening at the same time; he describes the heat of the dye and the expanding of the arteries. Of course, they often are done separately, not always together, but who knows that except for folks who have undergone one or the other? I certainly didn't when I read it the first time. Updike wouldn't want to put his reader through the repetition of two similar procedures. Or bother with the difficulty it would take to make them different. Updike's Rabbit character sees too much and not enough. One doesn't get as good a look at the monitors, even if they are unscreened from the patient. They swing around, and one's head is flat on the table, so one's sweep of vision is very limited. Someone viewing it could see a lot, but the patient sees far, far less.

Updike also has his cardiologist stand by during the procedure so someone can act as narrator, tell Rabbit what is happening: "Now comes the tricky part." Novelists are always looking for helpful devices, and this one, at first, didn't seem too strained. But there's always the question of a cardiologist who is not doing anything and yet takes the time to observe what Updike calls, inaccurately, a three-and-a-half-hour procedure. Whom would he bill? For what?

Rabbit's cardiologist tries to sell him on having a bypass operation right away, instead of down the road. That doubtless would have been good advice to take where Rabbit was concerned (he has a not-quite-killing MI at the end of the novel, but he is still barely alive when it concludes, and I waited for Updike's next installment, *Rabbit Rots;* I was disappointed when the more appropriately titled *Rabbit Remembered* was released in 2000).

My cardiologist had been sunny about the prospect of my angioplasty, saying, if it didn't work, we'd "just do it again."

That is because cardiologists can do those procedures. As mentioned, bypass surgery is done by surgeons, and, unless you are a cardiologist and a surgeon, you won't be doing them, or, more to the point, you won't be paid to do them.

In Updike's version of Rabbit's procedure, as in mine, the balloon is expanded twice, and Rabbit thinks, or rather sees and relates, "The tense insufflation repeats, and so do the images on the TV screen, silent like the bumping of molecules under the microscope on a nature program. . . ." Well, take it from me, neither Rabbit nor I thought, "the tense insufflation repeats." That word would have been in neither of our vocabularies, just like "reperfusion," that word I only heard after I had that truly rare experience—the one that lifted me out of the bed when the tPA busted through the clot. The event that was unmistakably pain, one you can only have in your heart after a clot is broken through and there is still live muscle tissue on the receiving end to feel it. It's no charley horse.

I was given and took home the device that did the angioplasty, since, like so much in modern medicine, it is a one-use mechanism.

It looks like the most delicate rotor-rooter, a device for cleaning out pipes. A thin nylon filament spiraling out of a plastic handle, an angler's device for the most elusive fish.

There is no need to construct, as Detroit used to (and still does) make its cars, an object of planned obsolescence, since they use it only once. Germs, etc. Shades of my first encounter with anything medically invasive, as when I brought home my tonsils and adenoids in that little brown bottle.

A few years ago, thanks to ever-expanding technology and the interest embedded in the demographics of care, I saw on TV my heart attack reenacted via computers and documentary footage. It's always amazing to have life caught up with, and surpassed, by technology. There it was in living color, the exact hemorrhaging into plaque. It was even in the same part of the heart. Computer imaged and animated.

I suppose the first time this had an effect on culture was with Masters and Johnson, when they made a clear plastic penis and filmed what a vagina looked like during orgasm. Their trail blazing was decades ago, but what it pointed to was the fact that everything the body did, or does, was going to be, sooner or later, captured on film. This is both reassuring and alarming.

And, after I had been on the Ornish-inspired diet (slightly modified from the original), I got to see Ornish himself and his original batch of subjects going through the trials of his experiment in a "Nova" program on PBS. No drugs, just diet. It was called "Avoiding the Surgeon's Knife." It asked the question: could atherosclerosis be reversed?

Again, there had been any number of precedents for this public exposure of the exterior of the body (rather than the interior), the Loud family PBS series ("An American Family," 1973) being one of the first, but now practically any group one could name has allowed cameras to follow along as their lives are led, however strange or wondrous or boring those might be. The medicalization of these documentaries has become fairly complete. Sex reassignment, reconstructive surgeries of all sorts, everything is beating its way onto film, for instructional or entertainment purposes. Now, there is even a cable channel where you can watch veterinary surgery and only veterinary surgery. Different cable systems have a medical cable channel devoted to humans, but ours only shows us animals.

(Thanks to Bill Moyers, I was able to see my former brother-in-law, the physician married to my older sister, die on PBS [in the first installment of "On Our Own Terms: Moyers on Dying," which aired in September 2000]. I know how much fiction one can find in the so-called nonfiction documentary form. It's not what you say; it's what you don't say. And Moyers left out a lot.)

The Dr. Dean Ornish documentary was particularly interesting to me, as I saw it a couple months after my heart attack. But a number of scenes stood out. His group of subjects all seemed to be male. Most were married, or, at least, all seemed to be hooked up with a significant other. The effect was an encounter group, since they came together over a period of time. Like a similar documentary about some young folks entering Harvard Medical School, the variety of personalities began to assert themselves. In the medical school documentary, the fellow who was the most aggravating, who got married during medical school and then divorced (the film makers followed them over the course of their early careers), was more or less led by his professors into anesthesiology, just so he would be dealing mostly with unconscious patients.

The one who stood out in the Ornish documentary was different, but just as singular: a very tightly wound guy, mad for exercise, not in the least overweight, who was driven to beat the computer installed in his gym's rowing machine. He had some strained relationship with his female significant other and was far from ever looking relaxed. When Ornish would push the meditation side of his treatment, the guy would not look overly convinced.

If a viewer was going to pick the person who was going to die in the course of the documentary, it would be this guy, and he did. When his death is announced to the remaining subjects (the last shot we have seen of the thin and fit-seeming fellow is the poor guy coming back from a run, where he tries and succeeds to outrace his significant other), Ornish can be heard saying to someone in the group that the fellow "hemorrhaged into plaque," which, since that was my MI's description, sounded too pertinent. But I didn't see myself in the personality of the man who died. I was—am—no workaholic, or obsessive about much of anything. If I shared something, it was a mordant viewpoint, but I have always found it rather easy to laugh, and, if permitted, I certainly can relax. That was my self-assessment at the time I saw the show.

A few years after Ornish made a splash, I was reading *Publishers Weekly*, the trade organ of the publishing industry, and there was a small article on people who looked after authors on book tours. Two such employees were quoted about the most difficult authors they had encountered. One said it was a guy named Ornish, and the story was: they were rushing to get to the airport, and she was helping him get his luggage out of the trunk, when he slammed the lid down on her head and she started to bleed. Ornish ran off, lest he miss his plane.

Doctors, unfortunately, don't so much become public intellectuals as much as public hucksters, though what Ornish sells might actually be good for you. In more recent articles, Ornish himself has claimed to have calmed down a bit, become less driven, though who knows if he has the genetic risk factors for heart disease.

I heard Peter Kramer, the author of *Listening to Prozac*, interviewed on NPR, and when he was asked if he had ever taken the drug that he was singing the praises of, he said no, he hadn't. I suppose there might be a problem there, another form of do as I say, not as I do.

There is a subset of current health literature written by doctors who become patients. The issues of empathy and sympathy are turned on their heads. Whatever variation of "Don't become emotionally involved" doctors learn, or adopt, is tested when the doctor becomes a patient.

And they usually get the most marquee-laden doctors' attention, far from the normal experience, such as mine. As mentioned earlier, Norman Cousins's 1983 book, *The Healing Heart,* suffers from this, too, since Cousins, though not a physician, was on the faculty of UCLA's medial school when he had his heart attack. Cousins's experience was decidedly atypical.

My original cardiologist once said to me as an aside during an appointment, "If stress caused heart disease, we would all be dead," thereby, at least indirectly, acknowledging the stress his profession caused him, besides downplaying what some physicians see as an important causal element. He was the electrician in his group, and so my bias would see him as more of a hard scientist. Unlike the more aggressive plumber cardiologist, who performed the angioplasty on me, the electrician was the one who urged caution, regardless of what the early tests (on the group's new machine!) were showing.

The effect of seeing cardiologists in a group is at least one version of getting a second opinion. They do have different points of view, which can be detected, even though they have inherent financial conflicts of interest.

Talking with my dermatologist (being a tenured academic living in a fairly small town, one can have medical relationships that do span a long time; I've had the same dentist and dermatologist for nearly two decades now), I alluded to my heart attack, and he said, "Yes, there is, like in childbirth, a lot of post-cardiac depression. You know, it should be part of the therapy that you see a psychologist. Who does that usually? The nurses? You could talk to your wife, but that's not the same. At least for a day or two, they should come by. You can't do much in two days, but it would be something."

The oddity of that conversation is that it took place nine years after my heart attack. At the time, my internist had said something along the lines of: A heart attack often brings up a lot of issues that if you feel you need to talk to someone about, you should. That was the extent of that side of treatment. But I do think that would be a helpful addition, since so little is written about it in the popular literature. Ornish, of course, stresses meditation and calming techniques, as do a number of short-term health clinic spas that have sprung up in recent years, but it should be met directly. And it wouldn't hurt to have some sort of professional encounter for the heart patient when he or she was still in the thrall of hospitalization.

The planet of New Age, holistic health maintenance is often in the same orbit as heart medicine. Though "lifestyle" often reigns in this galaxy, some of what is preached is within the realm of common sense.

In the spring of 2000, the mayor of Chicago, Richard Daley, went off to the hospital after experiencing vague chest pains and not-so-vague blood pressure of 210 over 110. According to the *Chicago Tribune* (April 4, 2000), Daley subsequently had an ultrasound echocardiogram and a bicycle stress test, as well as an angiogram. The mayor, the even more laconic son of the legendarily laconic Richard J. Daley of yore, hadn't had a checkup in ten years. His brother John said the mayor harbored an "aversion" to doctors. I wondered, when contemplating this, if this "c'est la vie" attitude came from being born Irish-Catholic in Chicago in the mid-forties, as I had been. Daley had the angiogram, a doctor was quoted, because of Daley's decade-long lack of contact with physicians. He was in the hospital, and in that case, "When the iron is hot, you grab it. . . . We had a captive audience and we kept him." It was reported that Daley was put on a blood pressure–lowering medicine, Altace. That seems prudent.

Following Daley's difficulties came the selection of Richard Cheney as the Republican vice presidential candidate for Campaign 2000. Immediately upon his ascendancy, articles appeared in most newspapers and magazines on Cheney's history of three (three!) heart attacks and subsequent bypass surgery. The Bush campaign released very little information on his past or his condition.

After the November 7 election, Cheney had what was called, finally, "a mild heart attack." He had been taken to George Washington Hospital in the middle of the night by the Secret Service and had a drive-through angioplasty with a stent inserted. As I wrote in the *Chicago Sun-Times* (November 28, 2000), he was in and out so quickly that, had he been hustled out of the hospital in that short of time by an HMO, there would have been hearings held on Capitol Hill. But he left as soon as possible for political expedience: to show no weakness. (Businesspeople and politicians are most affected by this. If the pack knows you are limping, it might turn on you and rip you apart. Academia is one of the few professions that doesn't consider hospitalization a verdict that you are damaged goods.)

In '91, when I had my angioplasty, stent insertion was fairly new and not yet widely practiced. But, in Cheney's case, nearly ten years later, it wasn't rare, but it wasn't medicine's finest moment to see so many of the staff of George Washington Hospital acting as if they were a Republican PR firm.

The press responded this time around with more articles, a bit more probing, and it was disclosed that Cheney's "ejection fraction" (a measure of the health of the heart muscle, a common indicator of the heart's overall health) was but 40 percent, not one to crow about (65 percent is normal). Dr. Michael Breen, also writing in the *Chicago Sun-Times* (December 10, 2000), offered, "The new thinking is that 95 percent of blockages happen suddenly—not over decades, but minutes." In any case, the vice president is the current reigning poster boy for life after heart trouble, in addition to being a champion of in-and-out hospitalization.

In early March 2001, Cheney returned to George Washington Hospital for another emergency angioplasty at the site of the stent implanted in November. Cheney has restenosis, recurring blood vessel blockage, which happens in 20 to 40 percent of cases. I recalled my worry for the first few months after my angioplasty that restenosis would occur. But it didn't. Once again, Cheney acted as if he was a role model for workaholics and was back at the job of shadow president the day after his procedure. He appears to want to make all other heart patients look like slackers. Though he does make some doctors happy, showing the world that angioplasties should be no more of a worry than a daily aspirin. Cheney has been their most effective salesman.

And, at the end of June 2001, Cheney again set a record for in-and-out time out of George Washington Hospital, having a defibrillator implanted in the morning and checking out in the late afternoon. That device, a cardioverter defibrillator, will quell a racing arrhythmia. Or so one hopes.[1] One reason Dick Cheney was able to run in and out in record time was that the doctors were waiting for him. As the rest of us know, that's not usual. But the vice president continues to make most heart patients look like malingerers.

In my case, the period of hospitalization gave physicians options. If Cheney had a pesky infection, he might not have bolted so fast. Yet I went, it seemed, quite rapidly enough, from a fully escorted environment to unsupervised home life.

CHAPTER TEN

Bypass

I know only a few people who have had a heart attack like mine (that 50 percent problem: only half who do are alive). But I know more who have had bypass surgery, or a heart attack and bypass surgery. Two of my brothers, my mother, my father-in-law, friends, and acquaintances. It did seem to become the surgery of the century's end.

In 1979, 100,000 bypasses were done; in 1989, 260,000. From 1979 to 2002 the number of cardiovascular operations and procedures increased 470 percent; in 2002, the American Heart Association reports, 515,000 bypasses were performed on 306,000 patients. One of them, in 1999, was my youngest brother, Brian, still in his thirties, thirty-eight to be exact. Another was my father-in-law, in his mid-sixties. Three years before Brian's operation, in 1996, another brother, Terry, then forty-two, had a quadruple bypass.

Brian had looked like he might need one; he had been an athlete (football) in his youth, but, as he got older, he kept on the weight and got out of shape. He had the typical O'Rourke diet of death, as well as a number of young children, a mother-in-law whom he and his wife took care of while she was dying of cancer, along with a hard job and plenty of stress. And those Slavic genetics.

The funeral of my aunt in Chicago in 1983, as recounted earlier, had brought the whole family together, and we certainly brought up the subject of our family's health, all pledging to do something about it. Less salt! More exercise! But Terry wasn't overweight and it looked like he did exercise, so in his case it appeared, after the fact, that it had been—more or less—straight genes.

Brian had both the look and the genes. To have a bypass in your thirties is to have it far too soon. My mother had hers in '83, but she was fifty-nine then and, after a triple bypass following her heart attack, is still alive today.

She had been suffering from angina for six months to a year before her MI, she recalled, when I finally "interviewed" her for this book. The angina had been what she described as dull pain, a poking, as she had with bad headaches, for which she took aspirin. My parents were at their lake house for the weekend when the heart attack hit: the angina symptoms, plus shoulder pain, radiating down the arm. The small hospital at the Lake of the Ozarks treated her for the MI, but a few days later she was sent by ambulance to a hospital in Kansas City for further treatment, which culminated in a triple bypass.

I had flown in from South Bend for that. Evidently, the MI just ran its course; no tPA in '83. Her current health insurance has a cap for drugs, and she has been on Lipitor for the last two years, along with Diazem. Her old doctor retired without telling her, and she has found a new physician who is worried about her high liver numbers. She gave up smoking before the heart attack (just) but has resumed drinking.

It was eight weeks after her operation that she had the phone call with her sister, Colette; a few days later Colette dropped dead in Marshall Field's. Colette had her first heart attack in 1972; her brother Jack had a bypass in 1988, the same year brother Joe died from his heart attack, out of the ambulance's rapid response range. Jack died in 1994.

I have a very melancholy picture of my mother and her brothers and sisters, Ralph's children, three girls and two boys, looking, as they are, were, lovely and intelligent, serious and reflective. They were born not many years apart, and in the photo they all look as if they are around twenty, a few older, the rest just a bit younger. Today, they're all dead, except for my mother. Aunt Freddy, who was a Loretto nun, died after being comatose for two years from a stroke, at a convent in Wheaton, Illinois. When we visited her for the last time, Teresa said to me, as I stood looking at her unresponsive, though breathing, body, "Touch her, talk to her, so she'll know you're here," though, of course, my then-brother-in-law the doctor had advised, if anything was going on in her head, it was random electrical charges.

I discovered recently my parents are participating in a long-term study on aging conducted by the University of Michigan, filling out elaborate forms, so their history will affect statistics to come. They are also, coincidentally, a Nielsen family, registering their tastes in television shows for all Americans.

Because of this history, my brother Kevin, the only boy without heart problems, went in 1996 for thallium tests after Terry's experience, though his regular internist had not recommended he do so. He just took himself to a cardiologist to do a workup. Kevin is the healthiest brother in any number of ways. He had a series of thallium tests and blood work that resulted in this appraisal: "The combined test findings indicate a very low likelihood for the presence of angiographically significant coronary artery disease." He had the same tests done again in 1999 with the same results.

Brian, in his late thirties, before his bypass, was having episodes of shortness of breath—sometimes bad enough to stop what he was doing. At night he often felt as if he had a slightly a-geometric "rectangular square weight" on his chest. He went to his doctor and was diagnosed with asthma. He was given a echocardiogram, which didn't alarm anyone, and he was treated further for reflux for one and a half years. It was then decided he had exercise-induced asthma.

Brian, given the family history, was 99 percent sure it was his heart. His physician told him sternly, "You're just having anxiety."

After having about fifty episodes of pain, ten of them bad ones, he said, he got a thallium test.

He quickly had a quintuple bypass operation, two years after he had first begun to have symptoms. His wife, Erin, though, on her doctor's advice, delayed for a week the delivery by cesarean section of their fifth child, so they both wouldn't be in hospital beds at the same time. Brian's heart surgeon had been a teammate on his high school football team, so he worked Brian in on a day the surgeon did seven operations. The fifth artery bypass was, according to Brian's account, "an extra," just in case, but one that did not "take," meaning, who knows. No blood flow, but the other four seem to be working.

Terry, who had his bypass operation three years before Brian's (and had been all the evidence Brian had needed to think his difficulties with breathing were heart-related) had first felt serious symptoms walking across Arrowhead parking lot for a Kansas City Chiefs football game (something that seems to run in the family, the football game connection). His seats were on the stadium's third level. He felt bad, and his breath, he said, was hot. The next day he was taking a walk with his wife, and he told her they needed to slow down. That evening during a weekly poker game with his buddies, he felt as if someone was holding his arms back behind him. He felt pain going down his arm.

The next day he had an angiogram and then was scheduled for bypass. A quadruple CABG (doctor's shorthand—pronounced "cabbage"—for coronary artery bypass surgery) was performed. Terry claimed he had only felt fifteen seconds of pain (the arms behind the back feeling) throughout the whole ordeal, including the operation. The diagnosis, he reported, was bad angina, no MI. He was forty-two when he had his bypass. Two years before, at forty, he had had a complete physical. His physician, after all the tests had been done, said to him, "You can go out and abuse your body any way you want to."

Doctors say the damnedest things.

One thing the three of us seem to have in common, besides the DNA, was that we were all at our heaviest. Terry, who never looked particularly overweight, was, for him, the heaviest weight he had ever been, 175. Brian was at his top weight, 247. And, I, of course, at the time, was at mine, too, 203. So that would be one good piece of advice to impart: if you are at your top weight, in other words, weigh the most you ever have—and have other risk factors—you better lose ten pounds as soon as possible.

I tried to talk to my brothers about the more existential aspects of their ordeals, the mortality questions that flood upon one, but, being my brothers and like me, they weren't overly forthcoming. Terry did say he found himself much more content to be just "William's dad." He, like myself, has only one child, a boy, though he got married fairly young, and William is now a teenager.

Brian was given a video on his surgery to take home to watch (not his operation, but a typical bypass), and he couldn't bring himself to watch it. But one of his daughters, Caitlin, did. She said to him, "That was cool."

Brian and Terry would, as we talked, lapse into a quiet seriousness, and their eyes would take on a different cast: wise for their age.

Both of my brothers are now thinner than I have seen them since childhood, but it is painful to think of both of them having gone through "open chest" surgery (which is how I always thought of it, since they don't open the heart unless they are replacing a valve). Joseph Epstein, in his *New Yorker* account of his bypass, calls it that, too.

We talked over breakfast at a pancake house. Brian and Terry both ate pancakes, though I stuck to a vegetable omelette made with fake eggs.

⎯⋀⎯ One unknown fact that is most important, regarding heart attacks, is where you are when you have one. The oddest story I've heard recently is from a friend who described a mutual acquaintance's experience, a white male, age fifty-one. Sitting in first class on a Swiss Air flight in Zurich getting ready to take off for the States, the fellow, a news producer at CBS, was seized with chest pain. Swiss Air helicopered him to one of the best hospitals in the world, where it just so happened the chief heart physician in the land happened to be on call that day, and he received what my friend called "swell treatment." The story is not an illustration of how first class passengers of Swiss Air are treated, as it is about the luck of where you are: the day before the fellow was in Kosovo, and he wouldn't have been helicoptered anywhere there, except, perhaps the nearest MASH unit, and the outcome would likely have been different.

First class in Swiss Air on the ground in Zurich is a good place to be to have heart trouble, if you can arrange that; the Notre Dame stadium wasn't the worst place to be (an ambulance was there waiting). But that is what confronts people. The roll of the dice, in so many different ways, some geographic, if not biological.

A friend was in Machu Picchu, and he experienced "chest pains," climbing to the top of one of the ancient ruins. He flew back the next day to the Midwest, still in distress, and took aspirin and a good bit of liquor to get him through the plane ride and called his doctor when he arrived.

The doctor sent him immediately to the hospital, and tests were done, and he did appear to have had a minor heart attack. They kept him a couple of days for more tests, but did not do any procedures, just gave him medication for high blood pressure. Everyone commented on the elevation of Machu Picchu and the effects of his exertion climbing what seemed like endless steps. My friend is from New Orleans, an overweight African American man, fond of spicy, fatty foods and still overweight. He lives on.

Another acquaintance came home from the university, where he worked as an administrator, and plopped down in his easy chair and fell asleep. That morning, before work, he had been lifting weights with his teenage son, doing a hundred twenty-pound butterfly reps. He awoke and told his wife, a nurse, he was "feeling bad," that a pain was going down his arm. His wife said, "You're having a heart attack. Take two aspirin," and went to talk to her son, who was calling to her from the kitchen. He fell back asleep. His wife, telling me the story, then said in exasperation, "What person falls asleep while having a heart attack?"

She awakened her husband and asked him if he had taken the aspirin, and he said he couldn't find them. She said, again, to me in exasperation, "Isn't that just like a man?"

Yes, it's just like years of gender stereotyping playing out perfectly, that's for sure.

They finally got him to the hospital. In his case, nitroglycerin helped. He had been, all his life, an exercise fanatic, and though his arteries were badly blocked (LAD 40 to 50 percent, right artery thoroughly blocked), he had developed many collaterals, and they were taking up the slack. He did have the usual bad family history, but he is now only taking a beta-blocker and Lipitor. He continues to exercise mightily.

And there are so many sad cases, the other side of the 50 percent. One that struck home was the death of Kevin McAuliffe, since it seemed to involve literary disappointment. He had put together a book, the *Sayings of Generalissimo Giuliani*, quotations from the mayor of New York City with commentary by McAuliffe. Rudy Giuliani was to run against Hillary Clinton for Senator from New York, and the book was expected to do well. The day McAuliffe's book was published, Giuliani dropped out of the race for his own medical reasons (along with some domestic ones). I can understand the disappointment McAuliffe must have felt. A week later he died of a heart attack in a Manhattan movie theater, watching a matinee. I asked a mutual friend what movie McAuliffe had been watching, but he said he didn't know and no one had asked.

My own heart attack, as mentioned, inspired at least one bypass operation, my colleague's husband. Bypasses are so usual these days, they are letting machines, robotics, do them. When any procedure becomes run of the mill, ways to automate it will follow. One of the eerie possibilities is that the surgeon now need not be in the same location, city, or country as the patient. It is specialization at its most intense. One surgeon sitting like the Wizard of Oz, nudging the controls far, far way, of many patients in many places. The day, as they say, will come (*New York Times*, April 4, 2000).

I saw a bit of David Letterman's February 21, 2000, show, the night he returned to the air after having his bypass operation. During the evening he brought out the entire surgical and nursing team that dealt with him while he was hospitalized. All the doctors and nurses lined up like bashful Rockettes in front of a curtain to Letterman's right. He didn't go over to them, but introduced them from his usual position, sitting behind a desk. He lavished a great deal of gratitude on them, but, by the end of his remarks, he broke down.

It was clear that he wasn't choked up merely because of his gratitude, but because he felt the cold wind of his own brush of mortality, the abyss. But, being a pro, he managed to compose himself and go on with the show.

Which, of course, is everyone's task who has had a heart attack or worse.

Bill Clinton brought himself back into the news with his bypass operation in the fall of 2004. On the "Good Morning America" television show (October 26, 2004), he told Diane Sawyer, "The number one thing I would say to people is if you've got a family history, you gotta be tested, tested, tested." The former president claimed he had "missed" all the early warning signs—though the general public was well aware of his many stops at fast-food joints and his love of Arkansas barbecue.

Unlike most pre-bypass candidates, Clinton had a personal trainer and was in good shape—"I worked out with a trainer. I was in the best shape of my life"—good enough shape to notice how short of breath he, on occasion, became. One episode was long enough to land him in the hospital, which resulted in his quadruple bypass operation. Public figures undergoing procedures are the pretext for a lot of information getting out in the media, so for a month readers and viewers were treated to instructional articles and pieces on the mechanics of bypass.

When my brother Terry had his bypass operation, it played a role in sending me back to St. Joe's emergency room. My parents had come to visit shortly after Terry's bypass operation, and we had Chinese food the first evening they arrived. The next morning (before going to an ND football game with my father!), I began to feel nauseous. The nausea was exactly the same sort I felt when I had my heart attack. Though I didn't have any other symptoms (other than paranoia, feeling faint), I decided to go to the emergency room, just in case. I had good insurance. My mother said, "What have I done to my children?!", meaning her genes, not that I was overreacting.

So my mother stayed behind with Joe. Teresa and my dad and I went off. I was clearly scared, which had taken over as the chief symptom. But I was willing to make a fool of myself. It had been seven years since my MI, and I hadn't felt this way since then. But there was no weakness, sweating, electric sensations, paleness. I knew I wasn't having an MI, but I let the similarity of the nausea and the fact that I continued to have good insurance outweigh that knowledge.

I walked into St. Joe's new emergency room, not the one I was wheeled into seven years before. A receptionist asked what I wanted, and my wife said, "He's having a heart attack," and they took me right back through the doorway.

I was hooked up to an EKG machine, and I began to feel better. The nausea had abated. The doctor was an Irish immigrant, not in the country long. Unlike the doctors of my first experience in the emergency room, he was quite forthright and full of conversation and concern. Of course, I wasn't having a heart attack. That might have helped his mood. Because my father engaged him in conversation, the doctor began to speak about Ireland. One remark stood out, "It was like a funeral, like they were dying," he said, about the immigrants of early time who came over to America. "Their parents would never see them again."

He advised me not to go to the football game that afternoon. But since my father had come to see the game, we did.

A year later, I was back in the emergency room with a gall bladder attack. Now that was painful! I was finally given some good drugs, and the pain lessened. The attack ceased, and my internist advised me to have my gall bladder removed. A side effect of Lopid, which I had been taking for eight years, was gall stones.

But I decided once a philosopher, twice a pervert. I wanted to wait for a second gall bladder attack before having it taken out. It is obvious even to me that my psychology regarding medical intervention has not changed that much, even with all the experience I've had with my heart.

Nonetheless, I suppose, if I am "lucky," I may eventually have a bypass too. (See the Addendum to the Afterword.) Though the current consensus seems to be heading toward the overuse school. Best I don't need one, though I wouldn't want to have another MI and fall on the bad side of 50 percent. The magic bullet of "statin" drugs is still being touted by their makers and in the popular press. One hopes; one wishes.

(I am now finally taking Lipitor. I had talked to my internist about the new statin drugs I had read about in the *Wall Street Journal* shortly after my heart attack in 1991. The *WSJ* is a good source for early medical news, since its audience is interested in what will make money, and, in order to make money, you need to know early what is hot and what is not. My internist wasn't interested in putting me on one of the new statin drugs. My cholesterol, because of my diet, had dropped to the low one hundreds. Pills were "poisons"; not enough studies had been done. Nine years later, enough studies had been done to convince him of their benefits—and my diet, not nearly as strict as the first few years, had raised my cholesterol count to right below 200.)

Even now, though, I still feel lucky. And the question I asked many years ago still haunts me: was my heart attack good for me? The answer, unfortunately, is yes. At least, I suppose, in the sense it was one I survived. If I had had one a few years later, it might have been fatal. And, the heart attack did change me, my ways. Perhaps not as much as it should have, but enough to keep me alive and present me with the gift of all these extra years.

Afterword

I recently asked my wife's brother, a newly minted doctor, why I didn't die.

He said it was chance, having to do with where the infarction is, whether it's near a sinus node, one of the two spots that regulate the heart's electricity. And whether you have sufficient blood flow to other parts of the heart. In my case, it appeared that both things were in effect. The blockage wasn't near a sinus node, and I had enough blood flow to the rest of the heart. He was flipping through my hospital records.

He offered that the heart is invisible, unlike, let's say, the hand. The amount of damage is hidden, whereas a hand's lack of mobility would be self-evident.

The hospital echo test of my heart showing how much blood is expelled was about 55 percent. Around sixty is normal, he said. That's why they called it "minor" damage.

I pointed out in my medical records the nurse's notes around the time of the tPA induced reperfusion. I wanted to know what "Bradycardic" meant.

"Slow heartbeat," he said.

And I wanted to know if the two events were linked. The tPA working being preceded by the slow heart rate.

No, he didn't think they were connected but coincidental.

He looked at the nurse's notes and the EKG record (whereupon the word "Bradycardic" was written) that accompanied it. I had read those sentences a lot since I had gotten the records: "1503. Comfort. L chest ache radiating down L arm to elbow. Pt. very pale, cold, diaphoretic. BP 87/26 HR 48. HOB lowered. Cool cloth to head."

It was 3:03 PM. I had been brought up to the CCU at 2:45. I had been admitted to the hospital at around 12:50. I remember the nurse putting the washcloth to my head, the Head of Bed (HOB) being lowered. I was, it was clear, fading fast. I had first encountered the word "Bradycardic" when reading the report of a man who had died of a heart attack. The Bradycardic episode happened right before he died.

But, in my case, the tPA worked at that moment. The next nurse's notes came five minutes later, at 3:08. "1508. Comfort—Pain lessening & B/P 108/62 & HR 67.Freq. PVC's noted @ present.

"1510. Cardiac output: Pt. more comfortable. B/P 124/79. HR stable in 60's."

I wanted my brother-in-law to tell me that the two events were connected, the getting worse and the getting better.

But, no. They weren't. He did say I was doing very poorly, and if I had been at his hospital, they would have brought me immediately to a CATH lab, or even bypass surgery, given me medicine to drive up my blood pressure. They don't use thrombolytic agents as much anymore.

"You were doing poorly," he said. He looked as if he couldn't bring himself to say, You looked like you were about to die.

In this world you want answers, but sometimes answers aren't forthcoming. And not just the answers you want to hear. Sometimes they just don't know the answers.

During a March 2001 press conference on Vice President Cheney's angioplasty following his episode of restenosis, a reporter asked the two doctors, why did it occur (meaning why did the restenosis occur)? Dr. Alan Wasserman, chair of the department of medicine at George Washington University, leaned over to his fellow doctor, Jonathan Reiner, and remarked, that's the "Nobel Prize" question. Both doctors chuckled.

On the radio later that day, I heard another doctor, not one of Cheney's crew, but just an expert giving an opinion, say, it was not so much a stressful job that caused problems, but just what an individual's psychological response to frustration was. That sounded right to me. There are all sorts of stress. Frustration, disappointment—they are a particularly potent form of stress. Many people I know seemed to have been beset with some sort of disappointment before their cardiac event.

Because of the vice president's condition and Bill Clinton's surgery—and the entire aging baby boom generation—the air has been, will be, filled with news of modern cardiac care. Cheney's defibrillator implanted after his 2001 angioplasty was the sort of device my doctors were considering for me in 1991, when they were testing their new machine and I was drinking too much coffee. Indeed, one reason Cheney may have been out so quickly after his earlier angioplasty, it appears, was because the sandbag phase of recovery from angioplasty has been shortened. The incision can now be done, it has been described, like a self-sealing tire after a puncture.[1]

Advances will continue to be made, especially if there is profit involved.

On the day of the March 2001 news conference with Cheney's doctors, I saw a television commercial: a man was in a hospital bed, and the paddles of an external defibrillator were being used to shock his heart. There were scenes of his life passing intercut with scenes of the defibrillator in use: his youth, his marriage, his work. What was this about? I wondered. There was a shot of him in a suit standing next to a copier. Finally, the punch line appeared: Don't spend your life waiting on the copying machine. It was a commercial for a photocopier.

And, not so long ago, my son, Joe, was at the kitchen table reading the signs of a heart attack from his Boy Scout Handbook. He read, in his sweet ten-year-old voice,

1. Uncomfortable pressure, squeezing, fullness, or pain in the center of the chest behind the breastbone. The feeling might spread to the shoulders, arms, and neck. It can last several minutes or longer, and it might come and go. It isn't always severe.

(Sharp, stabbing twinges of pain usually are not signs of heart attack.) 2. Unusual sweating—for instance, perspiring even though a room is cool. 3. Nausea—stomach distress with an urge to vomit. 4. Shortness of breath. 5. A feeling of weakness.

Yep, that's them, I said and smiled at him.

Your son wants to see you, I recalled, from that day almost over a decade ago. Yes, he does. Yes, he does.

July 2001–December 2004

Addendum to the Afterword

After this book was scheduled for publication, on February 8, 2005, I did have a bypass operation—a quintuple bypass operation. It came about in this way: I've been having two-a-year blood tests and a once-a-year examination by my internist. I hadn't seen a cardiologist for a few years, having gone from yearly treadmill stress tests, to every-other-year, then—after being assigned to a new, young cardiologist in the group—to not having any. He said, since I did regular exercise and had an office on a fourth floor and walked up many steps every weekday, stress tests weren't that important—or of much use, unless I detected some change in how I felt. At least, that is what I recall him saying. That was enough to let me let those tests slide. I no longer made yearly appointments with the cardiologist.

For the last few years I would find myself occasionally thinking what it would take to get a look at my arteries, to see how my disease, atherosclerosis, had progressed. A couple years earlier at a fund-raiser for my son's grammar school, I bid for a heart scan (a "Rapid Scan," Ultrafast Electron Beam Tomography) at a local hospital. I kept the certificate but never scheduled the test. A radiologist I knew said if I had a lot of calcium buildup, it would probably just show that.[1] Obviously, I wanted to know but didn't want to know. But this year, my internist noticed that the last stress test I had was five years ago. He suggested I have another one—this time, a nuclear stress test.

One was scheduled. It was the familiar treadmill test, with the addition of an injection of an isotope. I ran, hooked up to an EKG machine, a doctor observing, taking notes. After I stopped, he said it looked normal. Then I went to a room and had a picture taken of my heart, a lumbering X-ray sort of machine, which cranked around my prone body. A short time later, another series was taken, when I was at rest.

I did, evidently, pass the treadmill test, but the isotope imagery showed a problem. A few days later an angiogram was scheduled, with the possibility of having an angioplasty, if one was required. All of this had little of the drama of the first time I had the procedure fourteen years ago. But when my heart appeared on the monitor and dye was introduced into the arteries, the drama increased. "Look at all those blockages!" the young cardiologist who did the catheterization said. I looked vaguely at the picture on the screen, my heart and its arteries appearing somewhat lumpy, varicose vein–like. "You need a bypass operation! Anyone would tell you that!" He quit the room and went to go talk to my wife, and I was left to contemplate what he said in my Valium-induced state of calmness: What was implied in his "anyone" was a second or third opinion, if I was to insist on having them—or so I inferred.

Eventually, I was wheeled out to a recovery room, and an attending nurse, a male, put pressure on the groin punctures for some ten minutes or so and went away. No more sandbags. The new technique of rapid wound closure I had read about certainly worked. I was transferred back to the original examining room I had been in, and my wife appeared and told me what the cardiologist had told her. She had been able to see the video of the angiogram a number of times. While I had been in the cath lab, a name of a surgeon had been mentioned, a man whom the cardiologist recommended, and all the nurses spoke highly of him. I learned he was to come by shortly to discuss with me my having a bypass. The drugs I had been given for the angiogram were beginning to wear off, but the news of my needing a bypass had sent me into a distracted state: I was back on thin ice, in a state of vulnerability. The surgeon arrived, a slight, compact man. He said he concurred with my cardiologist and that I was a good candidate for bypass, fit—a word I was to hear a lot—not compromised by another heart attack, and would doubt-less have a "good outcome."

He had looked at the images from the angiogram and said he would likely be doing a quintuple bypass and thought he would use an artery from my left arm. He advised that there was sometimes minor nerve damage from extracting that artery, but arteries were preferable to leg veins. I had known that, so I said that I was happy for him to use the arm artery. We talked about scheduling the op-eration; I wanted to delay it a couple of weeks, given that Teresa and Joe had a lot of commitments coming up, and I needed to arrange things at the university. He said I was stable, so I could wait two weeks. That would bring us to the Monday after the Super Bowl. He suggested it be on the next day, Tuesday. I saw some benefit to that, meaning—given Super Bowl behavior—it best be done with a day's rest in between. Everyone would be more well rested. I did think it strange that both of my heart events were connected to football games.

~⋀⋎~ I had been asymptomatic, in so far I hadn't had any angina or shortness of breath previous to the catheterization. Fatigue is listed as a symptom, but given my life, with a younger wife and a fourteen-year-old, fatigue at fifty-nine seemed entirely warranted. My mother was fifty-nine when she had her bypass, and she is still alive twenty-two years later. That gave me some solace. Hers was a triple bypass, all veins. My two brothers, Brian and Terry, had their bypasses at ages thirty-eight and forty-two, respectively. If I wanted to look at my condition as a glass half full, I could conclude that all the medi-cal intervention and my changes in weight and diet had held off this outcome for fourteen years. And, most important, even though I had multiple 80 percent and greater blockages, I hadn't had another plaque rupture, no MI. The half-empty side was that I was stuck with the condition. Any chance at reversal only came about under the strictest diet and lifestyle changes—and it was clear I couldn't do the monastic work such changes required.

After some friends heard I was scheduled for a bypass, I was urged to look once more into less invasive medicine, lifestyle alterations. I was directed to the work of Dr. Julian Whitaker, a foe of bypass operations, and given a copy of his newsletter, *Health and Healing,* an issue that had come out after Bill Clinton's bypass. Dr. Whitaker had this to say: "What happened to Clinton was absurd. At the first sign of 'sawdust,' they just blasted away. . . . The data from the past quarter-century shows conclusively that bypasses do more harm than good for the majority of patients who submit to them."

Whitaker cites likely brain damage and other organ ills, that no effort was made to control Clinton's symptoms with medications, no lifestyle modifications suggested, nor nutritional supplementation offered. Well, that didn't jibe with what I knew about Clinton's case. Clinton had stopped taking his statin drugs on his own and certainly had been modifying his diet and exercise patterns (he had a personal trainer!) since he had left the presidency.

But I did contemplate that side of the fence, since I knew a lot about it. The days before the operation were not enjoyable, since I was having "faith-based" surgery: not feeling bad, I was taking their word (and the proof of the angiogram I had seen with my eyes), and based on the accumulated knowledge I had gained writing this book, along with the realities of my family history, I decided to roll the dice and go forward.

But, it led to bouts of gloomy contemplation. Teresa went to New York City for a job interview—the whole notion of which had been causing a lot of stress—and I dealt with Joe's many activities and thought of what was to come.

⎯⋀⎯ Most bypass surgeries are done under the cloak of crisis. Fewer are done in the atmosphere of elective surgery. So it was an odd period leading up to the date: I went in to the hospital for preliminary tests. One was to learn how to use a plastic device to regain lung function. My lungs, I was told, would be partially collapsed in order to make the heart more accessible to the surgeon. The technician praised how good my lungs were—a nonsmoker! she exclaimed—and said I wouldn't have any trouble restoring function. The device was similar to a child's plastic toy: you sucked out and blew in, raising a blue ball in a column scale. Another technician took "arterial" blood, a test I never had before, where a needle is inserted deeply (in the wrist), and this blood would be tested for a long list of ills—AIDS, hepatitis, etc.—and I also needed to sign paperwork that included permission to use blood transfusions, if necessary. The technician had an assistant with her, a trainee, a young woman, though not much younger than the tech. The technician did the procedure, but she had to do it again, since she didn't hit an artery on the first insertion, painful as it was.

In the usual harem profession manner, I had a male surgeon, and everyone else was female. There was the occasional male nurse, though they were few and far between at the hospital where the bypass was to take place.

The blood tech having to do the deep stick twice was an illustration of what I feared the most: human error. Given the complexity of a quintuple bypass operation, I pictured the many things that could go wrong. These weren't quieting thoughts.

I was given a bottle of liquid soap of which I was supposed to use half the night before the operation. I was to bring it with me when I came to the hospital, because I would be taking one more shower there. The lung technician had told me to bring the breathing device (I was to practice at home) back with me, also—or I would be charged for another one. I was told to tell the anesthesiologist that I had "situational anxiety," so I would be given some sort of Valium mix to calm me down while I was being prepped for the operation. That wouldn't be a stretch, since I was having plenty of anxiety.

—⋏— At home, I found myself in the grip of the last time syndrome: the last time I would . . . fill in the blank. Whether it be making love, drinking coffee, looking out the window, kissing Joe good night, it struck me as the date drew nearer that soon this might be the last time I do all this: Life. Death. One holds mortality at bay every day of existence, but when you have this sort of surgery scheduled you do latch onto the day, the hour, that they are going to stop your heart and hook you up to a machine and do what they do.

And what are you to say, the last thing to be said to Joe the night before the operation and the last thing to Teresa before I was rolled away into the operating room?

One tries to be optimistic, even if one is a pessimist—or at least I do. With Joe, I tried to be a bit upbeat. With Teresa I was more straightforward. When she asked how I felt, I said, "Scared to death." The cliché was meant to cut the sentiment, since I was feeling very ordinary things.

On February 8, I am to check into the hospital at five AM. Sleepless nights are a rarity with me, almost nonexistent. So I sleep a couple of hours and wake before four and use half the bottle of special soap. The only personal thing I bring to the hospital is my medical insurance card. Teresa needs to go back home to take Joe to school and will return right before I am wheeled into the operating room.

A nurse shaves me, a map of where incisions are to be made. She doesn't shave my left arm, and I tell her they are going to use an artery from there, but she said it isn't on my chart. I'm alarmed, since I want the fewest veins used, given the superiority of arteries for grafts. I talk her into shaving it in any case.

Then the shower and the other half of the antiseptic soap. Then I get a drip placed, and Teresa arrives, along with the anesthesiologist. I try to forget all the stories I've heard about that specialty. He tells me where I'll have various medical devises inserted, and as he is leaving, I ask for the situational anxiety injection. Yep, that's coming, he says, and adds that he only worries about patients who don't have any anxiety.

I have to take off my wedding ring: that's all that's left on me. It takes a while; some soap helps. Teresa says, Thank you for doing this, and I am puzzled momentarily, but, I realize, it means going through all this to make me better, to increase my chances of living longer. Or that is the hope. I say, I'll be back. Echoing "I love you's" follow.

⎯⋀⎯ The first thing I recall about coming back to consciousness was being unable to talk because of the tube in my throat but wanting to communicate: a pad of paper was put in front of me, and I tried to write out a few questions: "arm?", meaning did they take an artery from my arm as I hoped, and "how long on h&l?", meaning how long was I on the heart and lung machine. Teresa and a nurse were there trying to interpret my scratchings and provided what answers they knew. I went back under, though I did feel exhilarated that I was still alive.

The next thing I remember was having the tube pulled out of my throat: the graceful arc of an arm pulling in one motion, the long tube following behind. I was in a surgery recovery section. I knew if things were going well I would be moved tomorrow. I hadn't gone under general anesthesia since I had my tonsils out, and I'm sure the drugs now used are entirely different. One I discovered is for paralysis, another for unconsciousness. Teresa told me that the anesthesiologist told the staff to wait an hour after I woke up to pull the tube: it would take longer for the lungs to function by themselves. I dropped off to sleep easily and awoke when prompted. I knew I felt more intact than I expected. Being cut open, I presumed, would leave me feeling somewhat divided. But I felt intact. I remember that evening having one visitor, a friend, come by. I was twisting about, and the effect of the drugs was akin to truth serum, from what I can recall of the conversation.

Later in the evening, the Notre Dame men's basketball team was playing Boston College, which was undefeated late in the season, and I wanted to watch the game on television. I didn't have my glasses on, and the contest was hard to watch, but I attempted to concentrate when I could. Notre Dame won—as they did that USC football game fourteen years ago when I had my heart attack, a fact I found out only when I was researching this book.

In the morning, my surgeon came by. He checked the wounds, which had been bandaged. The arm wound was stitched, but fairly smooth. I wasn't stapled at the chest. I had no long incision in my left leg. They had taken a vein from my upper thigh, but had done it through laparoscopy, so there were just two smaller incisions behind the knee, in the back, stitched, and one near my groin, which had been glued. The drainage tubes were still in. "No one has taken these out?" he asked a nurse, then palpated my stomach and—surprise—pulled both of them out at once. They were both long, longer than I thought they could be, about the diameter of a garden hose.

The Swann device, which monitors the heart, inserted near the neck, was taken out later by a doctor's assistant, a new category for me, somewhere between a nurse and a doctor, in so far as she did procedures. She, too, pulled the apparatus out with a flourish, a number of wires. I was happy that all these things came out without a hitch, a tug, a tear.

─⋀─ Hospitalization, as a rule, isn't a pleasurable experience. I was moved from the recovery unit to the more general population, but I still had a single room. But no longer a single nurse. Many came and went during that period at all hours. I came in on a Tuesday and left on the following Saturday. The most difficult experience was to have a bowel movement before I left. The anesthesia had slowed me down almost everywhere. You needed to order your own food by phone from catering, a limited menu. But for those days it was a world of small pleasures: hot tea, hot coffee, even if it was decaf. I was having a standard recovery, but the elderly woman in the adjoining room wasn't: she couldn't swallow and had a raft of other difficulties, it seemed.

I was given hourly breathing treatments—many, at least—to improve my lung capacity. That did seem to be in deficit. I took pain medication, but the pain didn't seem to be overwhelming or, for that matter, bad. But, luckily, medical practice takes a more aggressive posture toward pain these days.

But I was alive, feeling intact, as I kept saying to people. I had a few visitors, but it was tiring being social. I didn't feel that the operation had reduced my intelligence—or had altered my personality. Would I know, in any case?

Indeed, I felt I had one distinct advantage over most people who have bypasses, at least an advantage over those whose bypasses were their first encounter with cardiac care and the specter of mortality it conjures up. That trauma had all happened fourteen years ago. I have a high anxiety quotient for first-time experiences; it drops precipitously for the second go-round.

$\sim\!\!\Lambda\!\!\sim$ At home, a friend had dropped off a Barcalounger in our front room. He had used it after his bypass operation as a bed and central resting place. The first night, since he had slept in it, I thought I would try it, thereby letting Teresa get a good night's sleep. I spent a restless night in it. The next, I decided to get back into bed, with many pillows holding me almost upright. When I left the hospital, I was given a heart-shaped pillow to use when I coughed. I was supposed to put pressure on my chest, so any episode of deep coughing wouldn't split me open. One nurse had said it has happened before, and "it isn't a pretty sight."

I lay in bed late at night, clutching my pillow, in a gesture that couldn't be taken for anything else than attempting to hold myself together. But I slept for a long time, more than in the hospital, where I had been awakened every two hours for one treatment or another. When I woke up after about six hours, I took more pain pills I had at my bedside and slept for another four.

It was more sleep than I had had for months. Joe's new high school schedule required us to get up at five o'clock, and five or six hours were the most sleep I had been getting for months. Teresa, that first night I returned to bed, didn't get much sleep. I hadn't dreamt much in the abbreviated sleep I had been getting, and any noise I made—and apparently my dreams produced many—woke her. My condition and operation had taken its toll on her too.

But for the next few weeks I got eight to ten hours of sleep, and it had its healing effect. I faithfully used the toy-like breathing apparatus that came back home with me, and once I got my lung capacity up past 2,000 (2,500 is the top of the scale), I began to feel better. I realized how much lung function dictates one's state of health. It took a week to get it up that high, two more weeks before I finally hit 2,500.

My recovery was uneventful—and given the circumstances, that's what you want: no events. The day after I got home, I finally took a shower, the first since the operation. I had been shown at the hospital how to clean the wounds and did that, though feeling odd about it. The left arm incision did leave a bit of nerve damage: it felt numb but with some feeling, a slight electrical effect, though that was concentrated on the top of my thumb down to the wrist. I hadn't had any loss of hand function at all.

—⋏— Recovery seems to be split into three segments of gradually longer time periods: two, four, and six months. Each segment is a plateau, and you do feel "better"—my problem was I was without any discernible symptoms, so the "better" I was trying to feel was only the state I had been before the operation. At three weeks I had an appointment with the surgeon. The incisions behind my knee were tender—and I feared infected. They were taking longer to heal, doubtless because the wound would bend when my knee bent. And I had noticed a small filament coming out of the arm incision. The stitches were supposed to be dissolvable, and this one hadn't dissolved.

My surgeon came in with his fancy laptop and inspected the wounds. Earlier an assistant had looked at them, taken a scissors, and snipped off the protruding arm incision stitch. My leg wound wasn't infected, it was decided. My surgeon said I could start to drive if I was off pain pills, which I had been for a few days.

And I could start rehab in another week or two. But I still shouldn't pick up more than five to ten pounds until two months had passed. A gallon of milk weighs about nine pounds, so we bought half gallons. Unlike during the period following the heart attack, I wasn't as paranoid about every twinge I felt. I felt better because I was still getting a lot of sleep at night, eight to ten hours.

I started going back to school, picking up the semester's work. Luckily, it was a light semester of teaching. I had colleagues cover the two classes I missed (it met every other week), and a former director of the writing program took over my duties for the weeks I missed. I had written two columns for the *Chicago Sun-Times* before the operation, and I had wanted to write one for the third week past the operation just to see if I could: it was my mental test, and I didn't detect anything harder than usual about the task.

‑‑‑‑ᐱ‑ I was ready for rehab and recalled how important it had been post-MI fourteen years ago. It's the feeling of being taken care of during the twelve weeks (the insurance limit) of supervised exercise. After my heart attack I went to the rehab unit that the cardiology group I was seeing ran. It was a small gym attached to their office building (which I have described earlier).

The new rehab was in the hospital. It had the same machines and many more treadmills. It followed a more extensive three-pronged approach: stress relief, diet, exercise.

I found myself in geezerdom. My schedule was flexible, and I was encouraged to take the long night class, since that is where most people who still worked were found. It conflicted with school events, however, so I took a time slot during the day. That put me with mainly retirees. It was about seven to one, male to female.[2] Most of the men resembled me and my relatives. Men with male-pattern baldness, heavy around the middle, sporting the bad fat—"brown" fat—that attaches to organs, that can't be removed with liposuction.[3] There were a couple of exceptions, but overall the men did seem to fit the pattern.

Here the nutritionist was very up-to-date, so much so she was in New Mexico attending some New Age–type confab on the benefits of raw foods and wouldn't be back for a couple of weeks.

This was a more elaborate model of rehabilitation, a version of a Harvard-based Cardiac Wellness program. I was given a loose-leaf binder full of information, entitled Self-Care. Its cover graphic was a square made out of words, all familiar concepts given my research:

Social Support, Exercise, Spirituality, Nutrition, Stress Management, Optimism, Reflection, Humor, Relaxation Response, Mindfulness, Emotional Healing, Coping.

For the exercise part, we were hooked up to EKG machines for the entire time we exercised, not just the first few weeks. We had a half hour of stretches, relaxation music, and class time, during which one of the nurses (it was all women, once again, taking care of the rehabbers) would go over the lesson of the day, culled from the loose-leaf Wellness volume, full of self-help psychological lore, a curriculum I had become familiar with over the course of my marriage, marriage counseling-"lite" as it was.

It was a form of group therapy, in so far as we were all in the same group: heart patients, post-event or post-op. Those with bypasses were the minority; most had had stents put in, multiple stents. Indeed, the last fourteen years had been a boom period for the procedure. No one referred to the operation as an angioplasty; no one talked about the balloon expanding. They used the word as a verb: "I got stented." It was that prevalent.

Stents had a better track record now, whereas fourteen years ago there was a large incidence of the device clogging up, so much so they weren't done regularly. But of late a new stent that was coated with anti-coagulants had come on the market, and it had a good record. So "stenting" was the norm. The rate of coronary stent insertion, the AHA reports, increased 147 percent between 1996 and 2000.

Indeed, had Dick Cheney had a bypass, instead of stents, there may have been more calls for his resignation, given the different perceptions of the procedures—though even bypasses are becoming, in the public's perception and in fact, more run-of-the-mill.

My doctor brother-in-law, Teresa's sibling, had emailed me some studies before the operation that bypasses had better results than multiple stenting—which wasn't even possible, in my case. While rehab was going on, these same studies made the popular press, and stories had appeared.

But almost all the folks in rehab were in the condition I was fourteen years ago. This was their first encounter with heart-related mortality. Most of them were treated because of a heart attack or symptoms that had driven them to emergency rooms. So they had the vulnerability of fresh experience, and the precariousness they felt was evident and, to me, familiar.

For some, their brush with death was a religious experience. One man assured our group he no longer feared death, since during his heart attack he saw a light—not white, but, for him, indescribable colors, and in that light was his sister who had died decades before. So he was prepared to die at any time since his destination was so peaceful. After he left the group, another elderly man who had joined us told a similar tale on his first day: he wasn't afraid of dying, since he had felt so at peace. At their age they seemed to have already passed through Elisabeth Kübler-Ross's five stages of grief and were ready to go. Popular culture may have supplied their white light imagery, but it was of help to them. Religion was highlighted as one stress reducer during our instructional sessions.

One comic moment came about when our nutritionist was pushing the benefits of Ezekiel 4:9 bread products. Two members of the group had looked up the biblical citation that is part of the bread company's name and began a discussion of its merits. It isn't flattering to the company, since it has to do with the preparation of the bread, not its contents. The argument is over whether it should be allowed to be made over the heat generated by human excrement, rather than animal excrement. That took the "healthy snack time" discussion in a different direction from what our overseers were hoping for.

I didn't feel like an interloper, but I did feel a bit apart, since I had the operation by choice—but only because the necessity was made apparent to me. But mixing with these older men and women (most in their seventies and eighties) made me feel I was being given a preview of assisted living, or what life would be like in an "old folks' home."

One of the "younger" men—he was in his sixties—was a member of a hula dance group, and he brought by his fellow performers, three elderly women and a slightly younger instructor. So the rehabbers watched the geriatric hula dancing, and I thought, This is what happens when you don't take good care of yourself.

But, of course, I did know I hadn't picked the right heart-friendly genetic pool, and I hadn't lived the healthiest life, nor had I developed a low-stress personality. But I could only applaud what the nurses at rehab were telling us all: to eat healthy foods, to exercise, to reduce stress—or to improve our response to stress. All this seemed familiar—I had written this book about it!—but I was happy enough to hear it all again.

We had two slide show lectures on nutrition and stress. I was a classic case of "irritable male syndrome," a Type D. Factors found in heart attacks were gone over. One combination was termed "Syndrome X." The nurse apologized for this being an old set of slides, though most of the material was accurate. Syndrome X has now become known as "metabolic syndrome"; it contains the four factors associated with Syndrome X: mild hypertension, elevated glucose levels, high triglycerides, and low levels of H.D.L. cholesterol.

Weight gain is a chief culprit in the syndrome. My syndrome was family history, hypertension, high triglycerides, H.D.L.s in the 40s, and "stress." It was depressing staring at the slide of Syndrome X. It's the same whenever you encounter yourself as just a statistic, one of a large group, an individual no longer, just someone who shares traits that make him or her likely to have what everyone else has.

The diet wars continue. Our nutritionist favors good fats, fears the bad, and any fat that is heated automatically becomes bad. So olive oil poured cold is fine; heated, it's a danger. White flour, processed foods, long lists of chemical additives, all to be avoided—as is sugar and sugar substitutes. It's all good sense, but she was fighting an uphill battle with the Hoosiers under her care.

But diets are big business, so big the June 2005 issue of *Consumer Reports* ranked them, from Atkins to the Zone. Try to do your best.

Inflammation is the new hot culprit in the heart world. The metabolic syndrome is accompanied by high levels of C-reactive protein, or CRP, a new test urged by a number of physicians in the field. My heart attack of fourteen years ago fits their model: fresh, or soft, plaque bursts (the plaque having triggered an inflammatory response), and voila: a blood clot forms.

Our lessons in the group room seemed a bit haphazard, but they would throw me into various past worlds as I considered the implications of the bits of information we all were being shown.

⎍⏜ Teresa was appalled at the sight of me in the Barcalounger, watching TV during the day. It brought to her mind how her father and her stepfather, both now dead, spent most of their time during their last years. Her father had died a couple of years earlier of multiple problems, though it was lung cancer that finished him. Her stepfather, too, had a number of problems, hepatitis and diabetes and general ill health. He was overweight in the manner of a lot of Midwesterners, and though he lived in Northern California, he was born and raised in Pennsylvania.

So my Barcalounger recovery condition was symbolic—actually, a specter—and she wanted me up and about as soon as possible. I thought I could watch some old movies, guilt-free. But I did what the rehab people told me to do, and Teresa and I took walks—or she shooed me out of the house to do so—and my recovery continued. She was happy when the Barcalounger left the house.

Again, I appeared lucky, in so far as no complications showed up. At this point, four months after the operation, I feel about as I felt before I knew I needed a bypass. My internist, the man who sent me for the stress test, told Teresa that I was one of those individuals who didn't seem to have pain nerves in my heart, since I never felt any angina before the heart attack fourteen years ago, and I didn't feel anything previous to the stress test and the bypass operation.

I took this secondhand news oddly. It translated into: So I don't feel heartache. That was news to me, but it was true: I never had any chest pain. Pain nerves in the heart do dull over time: the young do feel more heart pain than do the elderly.

The first two months I chafed under the weight restrictions, not being able to pick anything up. Joe began to fill in for a lot of the chores I had been doing. There is this period of invalidism: You feel like a patient. But rehab gets you out of that. It is reassuring to run on a treadmill (though it took a few weeks before I was "running") and have the electronic confirmation there was nothing wrong with your heart.

Given the healing incisions on my body, I began to feel empathy for those who had suffered gunshots or knife wounds. Every little twinge I had didn't alarm me the way they did after the heart attack and the angioplasty. Such an event does prompt an orgy of self-improvement, so restricting my diet didn't seem a problem. It took a couple of weeks for my appetite to come back. I didn't drink any alcohol for nearly two months. I wanted to resume being the person I knew, though I was glad that person had dropped ten pounds. I hoped to keep my weight down.

My sister Eileen, who had been a nurse, called—as did most of my family and friends—and she told me it would take nearly six weeks for the anesthesia to leave my body. I would feel better then. And I did, at six weeks, though her telling me that might have had a placebo effect. Poor Bill Clinton had to go back under the knife to remove blood and scar tissue (like an "orange rind" it was described) from a lung nearly six months after his operation. His body hadn't reabsorbed the fluid the way it was supposed to. A friend said, "That's what you get when you have the best doctors in the country!" Clinton describes in the Afterword of the paperback edition of his autobiography that he had angina and finally went to a doctor about it when he had an episode not associated with exercising. At this point, Clinton says he's still not 100 percent, though I have no idea what 100 percent would be for the former president.

My cardiologist told me, after I told him my mother had a bypass at fifty-nine (my age now) and was still alive twenty-two years later, that originally bypass operations were seen as a "quality of life" operation. Now they are seen as a life-extending procedure. I certainly hope so.

My father, who is in his early eighties, is showing the preliminary symptoms of what is lumped together under the diagnosis of Alzheimer's. All of his siblings have, or had, it to some degree. I joke with friends that with any luck the bypass will let me live long enough to get Alzheimer's. In the fourteen years since my heart attack, medicine has improved. My surgeon had been practicing at the hospital where I had my operation for fourteen years. I was happy for his experience. Who knows what another fourteen years will bring, in medicines or in life? I hope my spasm of self-improvement will continue, make it easier to eat well, exercise, take my meds, and try to relax.

As I wrote in chapter 10, I had thought it likely that I would have a bypass at some time. What I worried over would be the when and where. So I am grateful that the circumstances weren't dire and that it apparently has gone as well as such things can. In rehab, one common emotion is evident: all the participants are glad to be alive. No one goes to rehab who doesn't want that, and the resulting atmosphere is both supportive and serene. Here's to life.

June 6, 2005

Notes

chapter one   **Here's Mine**

1. According to the nurses' notes (I requested and got my medical records from the hospital a number of years after the attack), I was admitted to the CCU (critical care unit) at 1445 (2:45 PM) on October 26, 1991. The handwritten entry reads as follows: "45y/o male from ER with acute inferior MI. TPA, lidocaine, heparin infusing. Pt. alert and anxious. Wife with pt. Cont. to experience L chest ache and somewhat nauseated. Color pale." An EKG strip is taped below. Eighteen minutes later there is this entry: "L chest ache radiating down L arm to elbow. Pt. very pale, cold, diaphoretic. B/P down, 87/36, HR down 48. HOB lowered. Cool cloth to head."

I remember the cool cloth to my forehead. It is clear—at least to me—I was about to die. On the EKG strip pasted below the second entry is written "Bradycardic." (During the research for this book the only other time I encountered the word was in a medical report of a man's death by heart attack. He was "Bradycardic" right before death.) The pain I felt, which propelled me upright, was caused by the reperfusion of blood coming back into the dying heart muscle. The tPA had busted the clot, blood began to flow again, and the reperfusion lit me up. Blood flowing back into muscle is worse than a muscle cramping from being deprived of blood. The two events, the previous drop in my blood pressure and the tPA working, were not causal; they, fortunately, were coincidental. Five minutes later, there is this entry: "Pain lessening and B/P up 108/62 and HR 67. Freq. PVC's noted @ present." Two minutes later my blood pressure was up to 124/79. My heart rate was "stable in the 60's." The tPA had worked and none too soon. Twenty minutes later was the notation that my doctor was "notified of cont. pain and episode of brady—hypotension."

About two years later, I read in the local paper, the *South Bend Tribune* (May 2, 1993), that at the time I was admitted, St. Joseph's Hospital was conducting a study for GUSTO comparing tPA and streptokinase. The study was sponsored by Genentech, which controls the rights for tPA. It was supposed to be a double-blind study, but who was enrolled was discretionary. If I had been as indigent as I had looked, I might have been given the streptokinase, which is cheaper by far. That is why the cardiologist's decision to give me tPA seemed—even at the time—to be momentous, but not just for my general care, but because it kept me out of the study: I was no longer "randomized." St. Joseph's enrolled about fifty patients in the study.

chapter two   Connected to Time

1. Teresa spent a great deal of the time with me at the hospital. The nurses' notes are pertinent: "Wife here. Both pt. & wife teary-eyed. Pt. states 'I'm just depressed.' Valium 5mg p.o. given @0900. Talked @ great length with pt. & wife regarding their questions about TPA, cardiac care, previous & future life style, etc. Pt. states 'I feel I could have prevented some of this.' More relaxed with talking. . . . Pt. and wife talking great deal."

2. An angiogram (or angiography) is an invasive imaging procedure that usually involves inserting a catheter into an artery leading to the heart muscle or brain and injecting a radioactive tracer into the bloodstream via the catheter. Angioplasty is also an invasive procedure in which a catheter is inserted into a narrowed artery. A tiny balloon may be placed at the tip of the catheter; it is inflated in order to widen the vessel.

3. My mother's father, Ralph Kompare, was from Slovenia, the son of Joseph F. Kompare of Metlika, Slovenia, who died, as the account I found put it, "at the early age of 50." Joseph Kompare ran a saloon in South Chicago, which, according to the same account, was a clearing house for new Eastern European immigrants, often those brought to the saloon by "the police wagon." His son Ralph was "one of the first lawyers of Slovenian descent in the U.S."

4. From the nurses' notes:

I visited with Mr. O'Rourke and asked him how his stay has been. He related to me he was very upset by not being told he could be transferred and having to move at night. The move turned out to be smooth and he was able to sleep. I shared with Mr. O'Rourke CUI's intent on moving at 12 midnight. It was to secure him the private room on the floor which had been opened and move him at 12 while he was still awake rather than wait and gamble on no patient needing it during the night. I also assured the patient that it is our practice to inform the patient whenever we can to a lower activity unit. This was an oversight and the nurse will be reminded on how important this is to the patient to prepare for the move. Mr. O'Rourke was pleased with the follow-up.

Elsewhere in the nurses' notes around this time were remarks such as: "Does not speak unless spoken to. Does not make eye contact."

5. Tony Kerrigan didn't die directly from his heart problems, but from advanced prostate cancer. I discovered some years after he died the reason he wasn't given more streptokinase in the hospital when he had his second attack: they can only give you that thrombolytic once, whereas they can administer tPA more than once, which is why my doctor wanted me to have it.

6. From the doctor's notes: "This patient has focal high grade stenosis in the distal right coronary artery, with hemorrhage into a plaque. There is only a mild wall motion abnormality in the diaphragmatic wall. This lesion is high grade and in my opinion should probably be treated with Coronary Angioplasty after a few more days of Heparin."

chapter three   Infection

1. These event-based infections are testing the limits of antibiotics. Vancomycin was the drug of choice at the time.

2. I did two articles at the time of the controversy and one a year later, along with appearing on the radio and at public forums. See my book *Signs of the Literary Times: Essays, Reviews, Profiles 1970–1992* (Albany: State University of New York Press, 1993), 66–87.

3. From the doctor's notes:

The patient was taken to the Cath Lab. Both groins were prepped and draped. Under local 2% Xylocaine, I placed a long USCI 8 French sheath in the right femoral artery, and a 6 French sheath in the right femoral vein. Guiding Right Coronary Angiograms were performed initially with a JR4 guiding catheter, but then this was exchanged for a right Amplatz, and then a right Arani catheter in order to give me better back up. I had great difficulty passing a Hi-Torque Floppy wire through the lesion in the distal portion of the right coronary artery, and I had even greater difficulty trying to pass the Picoleno balloon catheter into this area. The vessel appeared to be diffusely diseased. Two balloon inflations up to only two atmospheres were performed at the site of the lesion. The lesion was soft and the balloon filled out well, and the vessel looked good on the video tape after those two inflations. There was an area that was felt to be probably spasm around the curve in the artery more proximally. This was unresponsive to Nitroglycerin given intracoronary, and therefore I treated that spasm also with balloon Angioplasty again to two atmospheres, with success. At the end of the procedure, the catheter and sheath was removed, and then repeat Angiography was performed. The patient had discomfort in his chest during each balloon inflation described as a heaviness or tightness, and at the end of the study he had an opened artery and no discomfort. . . . The final stenosis was about 30%.

chapter four   **After the Catheterization**

1. From the hospital records:

Hospital Course. The patient was admitted to Saint Joseph's Medical Center's Coronary Care Unit with an acute inferior wall myocardial infarction. DPL was started in the emergency room at a total of 100 mg. He was started on intravenous Lidocaine along with heparin and intravenous Nitroglycerin. There was evidence of reperfusion suggested by peaking CPK enzymes with a maximum CPK of 1,185 at 14% CPK MB. There was also evidence reperfusion arrhythmias following TPA infusion. The patient was maintained on intravenous heparin therapy.

During this stay he had elevation of temperature. There was evidence of infection in the IV site on the right wrist. Culture showed presence of staph aureus which was sensitive to Vancomycin. Initially before the cultures were available, the patient was treated with intravenous Cephalothin. Subsequently he was changed to Vancomycin because of continuous elevation temperature. The patient responded to antibiotic therapy well and had defervation of fever in a week's period of time.

His PTT time was maintained above 50 seconds. The patient was started on a calcium channel blocker in the form of Cardizem 50 mg p.o. q.8h. After the patient recovered from his fever, he underwent cardiac catheterization which showed evidence of 90% lesion in the mid-right coronary artery. Also evidence of black rupture which might have caused his infarction. Left ventricular function was fairly normal with very little evidence of inferior wall hypokinesis. After the patient was treated with antibiotics for about 7 days, he underwent angioplasty of his right coronary artery on 11-4-91. There were no complications following the angioplasty. The patient was discharged home on 11-6-91.

chapter five   A Shadow Biography

1. In December 1986 my cholesterol was 269 and my triglycerides 211, both high. A note next to the cholesterol reading was "HI ASHD Risk"—I was in the ninetieth percentile for my age. In August 1988 my readings were cholesterol 196 and triglycerides 137, after my small "lifestyle" and diet changes during those years.

chapter six   The Lucky Disease

1. Kathy Boudin was released in fall 2003 after serving twenty-two years.

chapter seven   In My Own House

1. I realize two of the most daunting problems concerning heart attacks are money and employment. In June 2004, Families USA released a report, "One in Three: Non-Elderly Americans without Health Insurance." Beyond that stark fact is the cost of post-treatment: the drugs I use, if not mostly covered by my health insurance, would take a big chunk of my disposable income. And my job, teaching at a university, allows for the most flexible adjustment post–heart attack of any I know. The New York Times ran a series of articles on class in America, and the second in the series described three different heart attacks (May 16, 2005). The upper-middle-class individual's experience seemed rather typical. The two other (middle- and lower-class) seemed somewhat exceptional: one was a worker who had three decades with a public utility and fairly decent health insurance; the lower-class individual was an Eastern European immigrant, with little English,

and she received very hit-and-miss care. The *Times'* coverage confirmed what most know, that health care is delivered unevenly throughout the country and our society. The *Times* took almost no notice of the role of chance and luck in the process.

chapter eight   The Medically Compromised

1. Current drug list below.
ASA (Ecotrin) 325 milligrams daily—anti-inflammatory
Atenolol 50 milligrams daily—beta-blocker
Lipitor 10 milligrams daily—statin
Zyrtec 10 milligrams daily—for allergies
Lisinopril 10 milligrams daily—ace inhibitor, blood pressure
Lopid 600 milligrams twice daily—to lower triglycerides
This is the preferred daily cocktail heart patients like me are on.

chapter nine   The Subject Turned to Health

1. During 2005, a number of reports appeared citing problems with this sort of device. See "Study Shows Increase in Defibrillator Defects," *USA Today,* September 19, 2005, 18A.

Afterword

1. See http://www.vascularsolutions.com. This site will show one method of rapid sealing. The internet has become the universal library, and search engines will take you anywhere and everywhere. WebMD.com is a place to start, but the sites are legion.

Addendum to the Afterword

1. *Time* magazine (September 5, 2005) calls calcium "The Newest Risk Factor" and devotes a number of pages to the technology that detects and measures it.
2. Cardiovascular disease is the number one killer of women in the United States, killing 500,000 every year. This is more than the next six

causes of death combined, according to Bayer MedicalCare. And in 2001 Yale-New Haven Hospital cited studies reporting middle-aged women are more likely to die within two years after a heart attack than men the same age.

3. Here is what physicians from Johns Hopkins University School of Medicine have to say about this sort of fat: "Fat is not an inert substance—it is an active organ. Among its harmful characteristics is the production of proteins called cytokines that promote inflammation and are associated with an increased risk of heart disease. Chronic inflammation can injure the lining of artery walls, making them susceptible to the accumulation of fatty plaque deposits that can ultimately rupture and cause a heart attack or stroke" (http://www.hopkinsmedicine.org).

The List

Every book of this sort should have a list. Here's mine.

1. There are a lot of danger signs for an impending heart attack. Here is one not often mentioned, but seems to run true: If you are at your top weight, meaning you weigh more now than you ever have, you are in danger. That is the straw that often breaks this camel's back. If you are at your heaviest, lose weight; even if you remain at the end overweight, you are at least not pushing your own personal envelope.
2. See above.
3. Everything they say about exercise is true. But you don't have to become a triathlete. Nonetheless, you cannot remain sedentary. Walk, if you don't want to run.
4. If you have family history, make sure your doctor knows of it, and take steps to counter its own hidden agenda.
5. Ditto high blood pressure.
6. Stress should be avoided for general health, but if you find you are in a particularly bad patch, and are generally worn down psychically, make sure your weight and blood pressure are not as high as you are low.
7. If you anger easily and have other risk factors, watch out.
8. Good spirits are overrated, but generosity never kills anyone.
9. Take your medicines.
10. Eat sensibly.

Glossary

ACE inhibitor (angiotensin-converting enzyme inhibitor): A category of drug used to treat high blood pressure and heart failure.

Acute myocardial infarction: An event caused by death of heart muscle due to obstruction or blockage of a coronary artery.

Aerobic exercise: Exercise characterized by repetitive movement of large muscle groups; the energy needed is supplied by inspired oxygen.

Aneurysm: A sac formed by the dilatation of the wall of an artery, a vein, or a heart chamber.

Angina pectoris: Pain or discomfort in the chest due to inadequacy of blood supply to meet oxygen demands of the myocardium, commonly precipitated by effort or emotion.

Angiographically significant CAD: A 70 percent or greater diameter blockage of one or more major epicardial coronary artery segments or a 50-percent diameter stenosis of the left main coronary artery shown by X-ray examination after injection of fluid opaque to X-rays. (*CAD:* See *Coronary artery disease.*)

Arrhythmia: Alteration of the normal rhythm of the heart; abnormal heart rhythm.

Atherosclerosis: A common form of arteriosclerosis in which yellowish plaques (atheromas) containing cholesterol, lipoid material, and lipophages form within or beneath the intima of large- and medium-size arteries.

Beta-blocker (beta-adrenergic blocking agent): A drug that antagonizes the effect of sympathetic stimulation, producing a decrease in heart rate, blood pressure, myocardial contractility, and stroke volume, and thereby lessens oxygen demand in the myocardium and decreases angina pectoris.

Blood pressure: The driving force that moves blood through the circulatory system. Systolic blood pressure is the blood pressure when the ventricular muscle contracts. Diastolic blood pressure is blood pressure when the ventricular muscle is relaxed between beats.

Bolus: A single large quantity of a substance, such as a dose of a drug, intended for therapeutic use.

Bradycardia: An abnormally slow heart rate. Also called bradyarrhythmia.

Cardiac catheterization: Passage of a catheter into the heart through a vein or artery, under X-ray control, used to diagnose cardiac abnormalities.

Cardiac mortality: Death due to disease of the heart.

Catheter: A slender, flexible tube.

Cholesterol: A lipid or fatty substance found in tissues or blood. Elevated levels in the blood predispose a person to atherosclerosis in the coronary and other arteries.

Coronary angiography: A diagnostic technique that involves the injection of fluid opaque to X-rays into the coronary arteries and heart chambers.

Coronary artery bypass graft surgery (CABG): Bypass of an obstructed coronary artery using an artery in the chest or a vein segment from the leg attached to the aorta.

Coronary artery disease (CAD): A progressive atherosclerotic narrowing of the coronary arteries with resultant reduction in the blood and oxygen supply to the heart muscle.

Coronary heart disease (CHD): Heart disease resulting from atherosclerotic coronary artery obstruction (CAD).

Echocardiography: Use of ultrasound to detect and record intracardiac structures and their motion and measure cardiac chamber size, shape, and wall thickness.

Ejection fraction: A measure of pumping action of the left ventricle of the heart, normally 65 +/- 8 percent; lower values indicate ventricular dysfunction. The difference between left ventricular end diastolic volume and left ventricular end systolic volume divided by left ventricular end diastolic volume.

Electrocardiogram (ECG or EKG): A graphic record of the electrical activity of the heart, obtained with an electrocardiograph.

Exercise test: A diagnostic test in which the patient exercises on a treadmill, bicycle, or other equipment with ECG and blood pressure monitoring, also referred to as a stress test.

Fibrillation: Chaotic rapid contraction or twitching of atrial or ventricular muscle.

Heart failure: Failure of the heart to maintain adequate flow of blood to the tissues.

Heart rate: Number of beats of the heart per minute.

High-density lipoprotein: A complex of lipid and protein molecules to transport cholesterol, also called "HDL." The cholesterol component that transports cholesterol to the liver for metabolism.

Homocysteine: An amino acid. High levels of homocysteine can raise cholesterol levels and contribute to the development of atherosclerosis.

Hypertension: Elevation of arterial blood pressure above normal range. Commonly called high blood pressure.

Hypotension: Abnormally low blood pressure.

Left ventricular function: Pumping function of the chamber supplying body circulation.

Lipid: Any of a variety of fat and fatlike substances characterized by being water-insoluble.

Low-density lipoprotein (LDL): A complex of lipid and protein molecules to transport cholesterol. The cholesterol component that transports cholesterol from the liver to the rest of the body.

Myocardial ischemia: Deficiency of blood supply to heart muscle.

Percutaneous transluminal coronary angioplasty (PTCA): An invasive procedure to enlarge the lumen of a narrowed coronary artery by balloon compression. The angioplasty catheter is inserted into a coronary artery, and the balloon is inflated at the site of an obstructing atheroma.

Radionuclide ventriculography: Assessment of cardiac chamber size and performance by intravenous radioisotope injection.

Reperfusion: The restoration of blood flow to an organ or tissue that is ischemic due to decrease in normal blood supply.

Restenosis: Stenosis, or narrowing, of an artery recurring after correction of the blockage.

Resuscitation: The restoration to life or consciousness of an individual showing no signs of life; it includes such measures as artificial respiration and cardiac massage.

Revascularization: The restoration of adequate blood supply, usually to heart muscle; CABG and PTCA are techniques of myocardial revascularization.

Risk factors: Characteristics associated with an increased rate of a subsequently occurring disease.

Stent: A wire-mesh tube inserted after balloon angioplasty that functions to support the arterial wall and keeps the vessel dilated.

Streptokinase: A drug that can dissolve blood clots; used to open obstructed coronary arteries in the early hours following myocardial infarction.

Tachycardia: Abnormally fast heart rate, greater than one hundred beats per minute.

Thrombolytic therapy: Pharmacologic agents designed to dissolve blood clots formed within the vascular system.

tPA (tissue-type plasminogen activator): A drug used to dissolve blood clots in an obstructed coronary artery in the early hours following myocardial infarction.

Triglycerides: A triester of glycerol with one, two, or three acid molecules.

Unstable angina: Chest pain of myocardial ischemia that occurs at rest, new onset of pain with exertion, or pain that has accelerated (more frequent, longer in duration, or lower in threshold).

Ventricular dysfunction: Abnormality of the pumping function of the ventricle.

Selected Bibliography

Books

American Heart Association. *Guide to Heart Attack: Treatment, Recovery, Prevention.* New York: Times Books, 1996.
———. *Heart Disease and Stroke Statistics.* 2005 Update. Dallas: American Heart Association, 2005.
———. *Your Heart: An Owner's Manual.* Englewood Cliffs, N.J.: Prentice Hall, 1995.
Arnot, M.D., Robert. *Dr. Bob Arnot's Guide to Turning Back the Clock.* Boston: Little, Brown, 1995.
Atkins, M.D., Robert C. *Dr. Atkins' New Diet Revolution.* New York: Avon Books, 1997.
Barnard, Christiaan, M.D. *Fifty Ways to a Healthy Heart.* London: Thorsons, 2001.
Benson, M.D., Herbert, with Eileen M. Stuart, RNC. *The Wellness Book.* New York: Simon & Schuster, 1992.
Biro, David. *One Hundred Days: My Unexpected Journey from Doctor to Patient.* New York: Pantheon, 2000.
Bolen, Jean Shinoda. *Close to the Bone: Life-Threatening Illness and the Search for Meaning.* New York: Scribner, 1996.
Bosker, M.D., Gideon. *Pills That Work; Pills That Don't.* New York: Harmony Books, 1997.
Boy Scout Handbook, The. 11th edition. Irving, Tex.: Boy Scouts of America, 1998.

Brandt, Nat. *Chicago Death Trap: The Iroquois Theatre Fire of 1903.* Carbondale: Southern Illinois University Press, 2003.

Brodkey, Harold. *This Wild Darkness: The Story of My Death.* New York: Metropolitan Books, 1996.

Budnick, Herbert N. *Heart to Heart: A Guide to the Psychological Aspects of Heart Disease.* Santa Fe, N.M.: Health Press, 1997.

Cleveland Clinic Heart Book. Ed. Eric J. Topol. New York: Hyperion, 2000.

Clinton, Bill. *My Life.* New York: Vintage Books, 2005.

Cooper, Kenneth H. *Running without Fear: How to Reduce the Risk of Heart Attack and Sudden Death during Aerobic Exercise.* New York: M. Evans, 1985.

Cortis, Bruno. *Heart Soul: A Psychological and Spiritual Guide to Preventing and Healing Heart Disease.* New York: Pocket Books, 1997.

Cousins, Norman. *Anatomy of an Illness as Perceived by the Patient.* New York: Bantam Books, 1979.

———. *The Healing Heart: Antidotes to Panic and Helplessness.* New York: W. W. Norton, 1983.

Epstein, Joseph. *Narcissus Leaves the Pool: Familiar Essays.* Boston: Houghton Mifflin, 1999.

Godwin, Gail. *Heart: A Personal Journey through Its Myths and Meanings.* New York: William Morrow, 2001.

Goleman, Daniel. *Emotional Intelligence.* New York: Bantam Books, 1995.

Gordon, Richard, ed. *The Literary Companion to Medicine: An Anthology of Prose and Poetry.* New York: St. Martin's, 1993.

Hackman, Sandra. *The Nova Reader.* New York: TV Books, 1999.

Heffernan, Deborah Daw. *An Arrow Through the Heart: One Woman's Story of Life, Love, and Surviving a Near-Fatal Heart Attack.* New York: The Free Press, 2002.

Hochman, Gloria. *Heart Bypass: What Every Patient Must Know.* New York: St. Martin's, 1982.

Klaidman, Stephen. *Saving the Heart: The Battle to Conquer Coronary Disease.* New York: Oxford University Press, 2000.

Korda, Michael. *Man to Man: Surviving Prostate Cancer.* New York: Random House, 1996.

Kramer, Mark. *Invasive Procedures: A Year in the World of Two Surgeons.* New York: Harper & Row, 1983.

Kramer, Peter D. *Against Depression.* New York: Viking, 2005.

———. *Listening to Prozac.* New York: Penguin Books, 1993.

Kübler-Ross, Elisabeth. *On Death and Dying.* New York: Scribner, 1997 [1969].

Lynch, James J. *The Broken Heart: The Medical Consequences of Loneliness.* New York: Basic Books, 1977.

Lynch, Thomas. *The Undertaking: Life Studies from the Dismal Trade.* New York: W. W. Norton, 1997.

Mason, Joseph W. *A Heart Attack Can Save Your Life.* Clovis, Calif.: Readers Choice, 1996.

McAuliffe, Kevin. *Sayings of Generalissimo Giuliani.* New York: Welcome Rain, 2000.

McDougall, John A. *The McDougall Program for a Healthy Heart: A Life-Saving Approach to Preventing and Treating Heart Disease.* New York: Dutton, 1996.

Moyers, Bill. *Healing and the Mind.* New York.: Doubleday, 1993.

Nordlicht, Scott M., Alan N. Weiss, and Philip A. Ludbrook. *Why Me? Approaching Coronary Heart Disease, Cardiac Catheterization, and Treatment Options from a Position of Strength* St. Louis: Northern Lights, 1997.

Nuland, Sherwin B. *The Wisdom of the Body.* New York: Alfred A. Knopf, 1997.

Ornish, Dean. *Dr. Dean Ornish's Program for Reversing Heart Disease: The Only System Scientifically Proven to Reverse Heart Disease without Drugs or Surgery.* New York: Random House, 1990.

———. *Love and Survival: The Scientific Basis for the Healing Power of Intimacy.* New York: HarperPerennial, 1999.

O'Rourke, William. *Notts.* New York: Marlowe, 1996.

———. *Signs of the Literary Times: Essays, Reviews, Profiles 1970–1992.* Albany: SUNY Press, 1993.

Osborn, Claudia L. *Over My Head: A Doctor's Own Story of Head Injury from the Inside Looking Out.* Kansas City, Mo.: Andrews McMeel, 1998 [1997].

Pearsall, Paul. *The Heart's Code: Tapping the Wisdom and Power of Our Heart Energy.* New York: Broadway Books, 1998.

Potempa, Sharon. *In a Heart Beat.* Seattle: Elfin Cove, 1998.

Rippe, M.D., James M. *The Healthy Heart for Dummies.* Foster City, Calif.: IDG Books, 2000.

Roth, Philip. *The Counterlife.* New York: Farrar, Straus, Giroux, 1986.

Salgo, M.D., Peter, with Joe Layden. *The Heart of the Matter: The Three Key Breakthroughs to Preventing Heart Attacks.* New York: William Morrow, 2004.

Speeding, Edward J. *Heart Attack: The Family Response at Home and in the Hospital.* New York: Tavistock, 1982.

Sprecher, Dennis. *What You Should Know about Triglycerides.* New York: Avon Books, 2000.

Stephenson, Larry W., with Jeffrey L. Rodengen. *State of the Heart: The Practical Guide to Your Heart and Heart Surgery.* Fort Lauderdale: Write Stuff, 1999.

Strong, Maggie. *Mainstay: For the Well Spouse of the Chronically Ill.* Northampton, Mass.: Bradford Books, 1997.

Styron, William. *Darkness Visible: A Memoir of Madness.* New York: Random House, 1990.

Superko, M.D., H. Robert, with Laura Tucker. *Before the Heart Attacks: A Revolutionary Approach to Detecting, Preventing, and Even Reversing Heart Disease.* Emmaus, Pa.: Rodale, 2003.

Tarnower, Herman, and Samm Sinclair Baker. *The Complete Scarsdale Medical Diet plus Dr. Tarnower's Lifetime Keep-Slim Program.* New York: Bantam Books, 1980.

Updike, John. *Licks of Love: Short Stories and a Sequel, "Rabbit Remembered."* New York: Alfred A. Knopf, 2000.

———. *Rabbit at Rest.* New York: Alfred A. Knopf, 1990.

Wegner, N. K., E. S. Froelicher, L. K. Smith, et al. *Cardiac Rehabilitation.* Clinical Practice Guideline No. 17. AHCPR Publication No. 96 0672. Rockville, Md.: U.S. Department of Health and Human Services, 1995.

Weingarten, Gene. *The Hypochondriac's Guide to Life and Death.* New York: Simon & Schuster, 1998.

Wolff, Geoffrey. *A Day at the Beach.* New York: Alfred A. Knopf, 1992.

Writing and Well-Being: TriQuarterly 75 (spring/summer 1989).

Articles

Bowman, Chris. "Clot-Busting Drugs Given Final Verdict." *The South Bend Tribune,* May 2, 1993, C1, C2.

Breen, M.D., Michael. "Bad News for Cheney." *Chicago Sun-Times,* December 10, 2000, 45A.

Brody, Jane. "Why Angry People Can't Control the Short Fuse." *The New York Times,* May 28, 2002, D7.

———. "Women Struggle for Parity of the Heart." *The New York Times,* April 12, 2005, D7.

Comarow, Avery. "Healing the Heart." *U.S. News & World Report,* March 13, 2000, 54–64.

Elias, Marilyn. "Depressed Need Walk around the Block." *USA Today,* March 6, 2000, D1.

————. "Good Mood Really Is Good Medicine." *Chicago Sun-Times,* March 7, 2003, 5.

"The End of Heart Disease." *U.S. News and World Report,* December 1, 2003, 36–69.

Golab, Art. "Coated Aspirin Found to Do Little for Stroke, Heart Risk." *Chicago Sun-Times,* February 17, 2003, 12.

Goodman, Emily Jane. "Without Warning." *New York,* June 20, 1988, 44–51.

Gupta, M.D., Sanjay. "Don't Ignore Heart-Attack Blues." *Time,* August 26, 2002, 71.

Hechinger, John. "The Growing Case for Heart Surgery." *The Wall Street Journal,* May 26, 2005, D1–2.

Hensley, Scott, and Ron Winslow. "Hypertension Report Disputes Earlier Study." *The Wall Street Journal,* February 13, 2003, B1, 8.

————. "A New Option for Fighting Cholesterol." *The Wall Street Journal,* July 14, 2004, D1–4.

Herz, Steve, and Lynn Allison. "Is Bill Clinton Dying?" *Globe,* January 24, 2005, 16, 17.

Kolata, Gina. "Gains on Heart Disease Leave More Survivors, and Questions." *The New York Times,* January 19, 2003, 1, 16.

————. "Next Up: Surgery by Remote Control." *The New York Times,* April 4, 2000, D1, 4.

————. "Studies Question Effectiveness of Artery-Opening Operations." *The New York Times,* March 21, 2004, A1, 15.

————. "Two Studies Suggest a Protein Has a Big Role in Heart Disease." *The New York Times,* January 6, 2005, A1, 20.

Lombardi, Kate Stone. "Clinton Thanks Staff at Hospital Where Ailment Was Diagnosed." *The New York Times,* December 24, 2004, A19.

Marcus, Amy Dockser. "Heart Surgeons Try Using the Power of Suggestion." *The Wall Street Journal,* February 10, 2004, D1, 4.

Miller, M.D., Michael Craig. "The Dangers of Chronic Distress." *Newsweek,* October 3, 2005, 58–59.

Noonan, David. "The Heart of the Matter." *Newsweek,* Special Issue, Fall/Winter 2001, 75–81.

Odorizzi, Irene. "Joseph from Metlika." *Zarja—The Dawn,* September/October 1976, 6–7, 14–15.

Page, Susan. "Pacemaker Won't Slow Cheney Down, Doctors Say." *USA Today,* July 2, 2001, 4A.

Park, Alice. "Do You Know Your Calcium Score?" *Time,* September 5, 2005, 71.

Parker-Pope, Tara. "Risk of Heart Attack Is Greater for Women Than They Realize." *The Wall Street Journal,* June 1, 2001, B1.

"Rating the Diets from Atkins to Zone." *Consumer Reports,* June 2005, 18–22.

Ritter, Jim. "FDA to OK Artery Stent with Anti-Clogging Drug." *Chicago Sun-Times,* March 3, 2003.

Rumbach, David. "Cold Medicine." *The South Bend Tribune,* March 5, 2003, C1, 2.

Scott, Janny. "Life at the Top in America Isn't Just Better, It's Longer." *The New York Times,* May 16, 2005, A1, 18, 19.

Squires, Sally. "Hearts and Minds." *The Washington Post,* July 24, 2001, HE10–17.

Stein, Rob. "Inflammation May Impair Heart as Much as Cholesterol." *The Washington Post,* January 6, 2005, A1.

Tarkan, Laurie. "Low Cholesterol? Don't Brag Yet." *The New York Times,* May 10, 2005, D5.

Van, Jon. "Roberts' Work on Cutting Edge." *Chicago Tribune,* May 14, 2001, sec.4, pp. 1, 4.

VandenWater, Judith. "Halting a Heart Attack: If Given in Time Clot-Dissolvers May Save Muscle." *St. Louis Post-Dispatch,* April 21, 1992, 1.

Verghese, Abraham. "Bypass Nation." *Talk,* March, 2000, 105–7, 154–55.

Washburn, Gary, and Jeremy Manier. "Tests Are All Negative, So Daley Goes Home." *Chicago Tribune,* April 4, 2000, 1, 20.

Whitaker, Julian. *Dr. Julian Whitaker's Health and Healing* [newsletter] 14, no. 11 (November 2004): 1–4.

Wolinsky, Howard. "Reporter's Brush with Death Holds Lessons for Life." *The Chicago Sun-Times,* March 28, 2005, 22.

Zehme, Bill. "Daveheart." *Esquire,* May 2000, 106–11, 155.

ON HAVING A HEART ATTACK
A Medical Memoir

WILLIAM O'ROURKE

"O'Rourke's book and its long description of having a heart attack may scare the bejesus out of you, but it certainly sheds a lot of light on the subject. His book is full of life—full of heart—and necessary reading for anyone who's ever thought twice about the tough organ that keeps us alive."
    —Malachy McCourt, author of *A Monk Swimming* and *Bush Lies in State*

"The story of William O'Rourke's heart attack is as compelling as a thriller because it *is* a thriller. As always, O'Rourke's prose is crisp, witty, and wholly original. The chronicle of his recovery demystifies a frightening illness, leaving a reader enlightened and, unexpectedly, cheered."
    —Valerie Sayers, author of *Brian Fever* and *Due East*

"In the first few pages of William O'Rourke's gripping book I learned what it feels like to have a heart attack and how the pressure or pleasure of daily events can keep us postponing the visit to the Emergency Room. Now, I tell myself, I'll be prepared even in the middle of the night or at a sports event. Thanks to my husband's many years of MS, I did have an idea of how important a good doctor, a ready wife or husband, an eagle eye for proceedings, and even chance can be in determining one's future—but the uninitiated in such mysteries will find *On Having a Heart Attack* to be full of first person insights."
    —Maggie Strong, author of *Mainstay: For the Well Spouse of the Chronically Ill*

"For anyone who has ever had a serious medical crisis, or been close to someone who has, William O'Rourke's book is essential reading. O'Rourke takes us on a fascinating, compelling journey into the literal and figurative heart of a gloriously full and fragile life. He illuminates much about our vitality and our mortality, and the ways in which fortune and modern medicine can collaborate in our individual and collective fates. This is a rich tale by a splendid story-teller—a most unforgettable, informative, and deeply moving memoir of one man's struggles and triumphs."
    —Jay Neugeboren, author of *Open Heart: A Patient's Story of Life-Saving Medicine and Life-Giving Friendship*

ABOUT THE AUTHOR

WILLIAM O'ROURKE is the author of *The Harrisburg 7 and the New Catholic Left; Signs of the Literary Times: Essays, Reviews, Profiles, 1970–1992; Campaign America '96: The View From the Couch; Campaign America 2000: The View From the Couch;* and the novels *The Meekness of Isaac, Idle Hands, Criminal Tendencies,* and *Notts.* He is a professor of English at the University of Notre Dame and the director of its graduate creative writing program. He wrote a weekly political column for the *Chicago Sun-Times* from 2001 until 2005.